Rahma SAID

Molecular deregulation in prostate cancer

Rahma SAID

Molecular deregulation in prostate cancer

Exploring molecular alterations contributing to the development of prostate cancer

ScienciaScripts

Imprint

Any brand names and product names mentioned in this book are subject to trademark, brand or patent protection and are trademarks or registered trademarks of their respective holders. The use of brand names, product names, common names, trade names, product descriptions etc. even without a particular marking in this work is in no way to be construed to mean that such names may be regarded as unrestricted in respect of trademark and brand protection legislation and could thus be used by anyone.

Cover image: www.ingimage.com

This book is a translation from the original published under ISBN 978-620-6-70198-9.

Publisher:
Sciencia Scripts
is a trademark of
Dodo Books Indian Ocean Ltd. and OmniScriptum S.R.L publishing group

120 High Road, East Finchley, London, N2 9ED, United Kingdom
Str. Armeneasca 28/1, office 1, Chisinau MD-2012, Republic of Moldova, Europe
Printed at: see last page
ISBN: 978-620-7-66443-6

Contents

Introduction

Cancer is a major public health problem, representing the second leading cause of death worldwide. Because of its impact on human health, cancer has been the subject of intensive research for many years. It is a multifactorial disease, involving both genetic and environmental factors. Prostate cancer is a cancer of the elderly, rarely appearing before the age of 50. It is the second most common cancer in men worldwide after lung cancer (Bray, Ferlay et al. 2018). In Tunisia, it ranks third in incidence among Men aged between 45 and over 85, with an incidence of 806 new cases/year (10.7%) (Bray, Ferlay et al. 2018). This cancer is characterized by slow development, limited spread and easy diagnosis based on several examinations such as digital rectal examination, Prostate Specific Antigen (PSA) assay and prostate biopsies. Its prognosis depends on age, associated diseases (comorbidities), clinical stage, Gleason grade or score and PSA level.

In addition to hormonal, environmental and genetic risk factors, the onset, development and spread of prostate tumors are multi-step processes regulated by numerous somatic genetic and epigenetic alterations, where molecular secrets are revealed by the tiny but powerful players that are microRNAs (miRs).

The present work is divided into two distinct parts. The first focuses on the analysis of Zeb-1 gene expression profiles in patients compared with a control group of healthy subjects, using RT-qPCR. The aim is to identify any correlation between expression levels of this gene and patients' clinico-pathological and epidemiological parameters, with a view to assessing the gene's prognostic value. In the second part, attention is focused on finding explanations for the deregulation of Zeb-1 gene expression, where appropriate, by exploring epigenetic mechanisms. This investigation involves quantifying the expression of three microRNAs (mir-548ac, mir-96-5p and mir-101-1) by reverse transcription and quantitative PCR (RT-qPCR), the latter having been previously identified as potentially targeted by Zeb-1 following an in silico study. An additional dimension of this research component is the association of the expression profiles of all the markers with the patients' clinico-pathological parameters.

Revue Bibliographique

A. Cancer from laprostate : Aspects epidemiological, clinical and pathophysiological aspects

I. Structure, function and histology of the prostate
I.1. Structure of the prostate

The prostate is a small gland of the male genital tract, 20 cm^3 in volume in the normal male state. It lies beneath the bladder, before the rectum and around the initial part of the urethra that conducts urine and semen outwards (Figure 1) (Lee, Akin-Olugbade et al. 2011). This chestnut-shaped gland contains several cell types: fibrous cells that maintain its glandular structure; muscular cells that regulate the flow of sperm and urine; and glandular cells that secrete the fluids to be ejaculated. In addition, it is formed of two lobes and surrounded by the muscles responsible for ejaculation and micturition, the nerve bundles located on either side of the prostate to control erectile function, the different duct to transport sperm from the testis to the seminal vesicles and the seminal vesicles located at each lobe producing sperm (Lee, Akin-Olugbade et al. 2011, Toivanen and Shen 2017). Furthermore, the prostate could be subdivided into different parts:

- The peripheral zone, which is the largest part of the prostate, palpable by digital rectal examination (DRE). The diagnosis of prostate cancer is made from this zone.

- The transitional zone, which surrounds a few centimetres of the urethra. The volume of this zone increases with age, and is where benign prostatic hyperplasia (BPH) develops.

- The central zone, which lies behind the transitional zone and surrounds the ejaculatory ducts that connect the seminal vesicles to the prostatic urethra. Very few prostate cancers originate in this zone.

- Fibromuscular stroma, made up of muscle fibers and fibrous connective tissue. It is a thickening of the apex surrounding the prostate. This zone contains no glands, so prostate cancer does not develop there (McNeal 1981, McNeal 1988) (Figure 2).

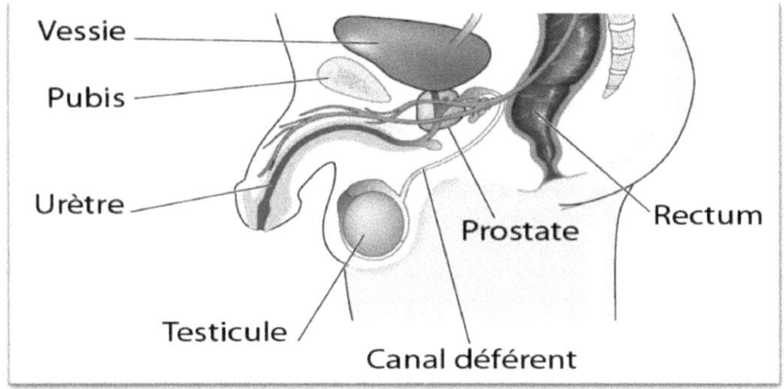

Figure 1 Structure of the prostate

(http://www.centre-europeen-prostate-paris.com/anatomie-physiologie-prostate.html)

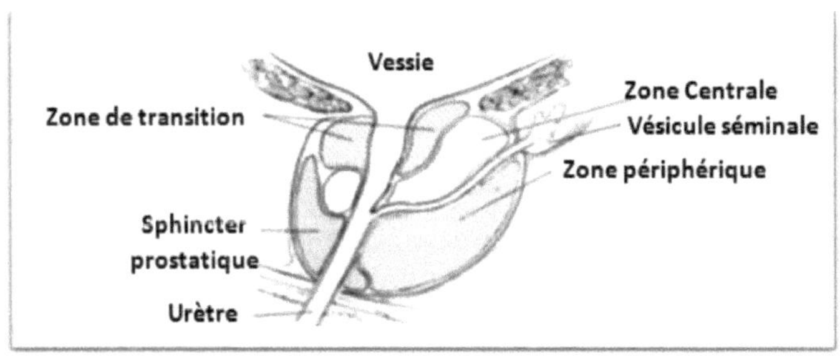

Figure 2: Male prostate anatomy

(Toivanen and Shen 2017)

I.2. Role of the prostate

The role of the prostate is to secrete a fluid rich in enzymes, proteins and minerals to protect and nourish the sperm. Following sexual arousal, the prostate pushes this fluid through ducts to the urethra, where it mixes with sperm and other fluids prior to ejaculation. This function is regulated by hormones such as testosterone and others secreted by the adrenal glands and pituitary gland (McNeal 1981, McNeal 1988).

II. Clinical and anatomopathological characteristics of prostate tumors

Prostate tumours can be benign or malignant. Benign tumors can neither spread throughout the body nor threaten the patient's life, and are referred to as benign prostatic hyperplasia, whereas malignant tumors are life-threatening cancers.

II.1. Benign prostatic hyperplasia (BPH)

Nodular hyperplasia or hypertrophy of the prostate is defined as an increase in the number and size of the peri-urethral glands, together with the supporting tissue. The increase in volume and weight (30-60 g) of the prostate forms nodules and creates a urinary obstruction. This condition is a benign process of the prostate and does not constitute a precancerous lesion. Microscopically, the hyperplasia may involve the smooth fibromuscular contingent (fibroleiomyomatous hyperplasia) or only the glandular contingent (adenomatous hyperplasia), or frequently both contingents (adeno-myomatous or musculo-glandular hyperplasia). The glands are always bordered by a double cell bed similar to a normal prostate (Briganti, Capitanio et al. 2009, Barry, Fowler et al. 2017).

II.2. Prostate cancer

II.2.1. Definition

Prostate cancer (PC) is the uncontrolled multiplication of abnormal "mutated" prostate cells. It is an adenocarcinoma in 95% of cases, developing from the glandular acini (Ludden and Jensen 1954). Adenocarcinomas are multifocal carcinomatous foci, often undetectable macroscopically, with the occasional appearance of white nodules in the posterior part of the prostate. However, there are other tumoral forms that develop from epithelial cells, such as intraductal carcinoma, ductal adenocarcinoma, urothelial carcinoma, mucinous carcinoma, neuroendocrine tumors and sarcomas (Hall, Nielsen et al. 1976, Vrubel, Mraz et al. 1979.

II.2.2. Epidemiology

Prostate cancer is the most common malignancy in developed countries, ranking among the top five cancers diagnosed in men with an incidence of 1.3 million new cases/year worldwide (13.5%) (Figure 3) (New Global Cancer Data: GLOBOCAN 201) (Siegel, Miller et al. 2017). Worldwide, this cancer is ranked among the top five causes of cancer mortality in men (representing 6.7% of total cancer mortality) (Figure 3) (New Global Cancer Data: GLOBOCAN 2018) (Siegel, Miller et al. 2017). In Tunisia, it ranks third in incidence among men aged between 45 and over 85, with an incidence of 806 new cases/year (10.7%) (New Global Cancer Data: GLOBOCAN 2018) (Figure 4). However, mortality from this cancer in men aged over 45 is estimated at 420 cases/year (7.4% of total cancer mortality) (New Global Cancer Data: GLOBOCAN 2018) (Figure 5).

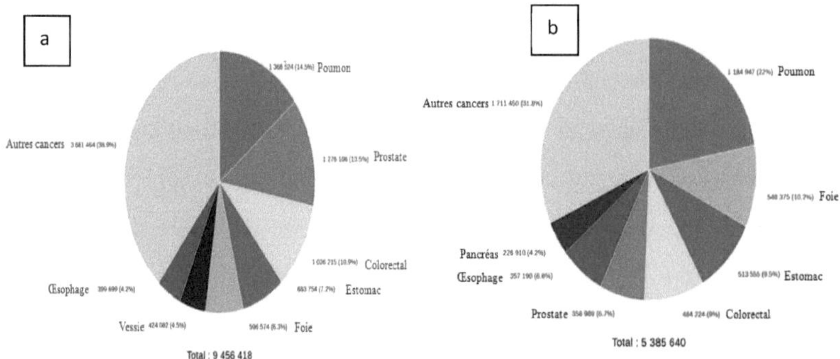

Figure 3: Worldwide incidence (a) and mortality (b) rates of prostate cancer in men (New Global Cancer Data: GLOBOCAN 2018.

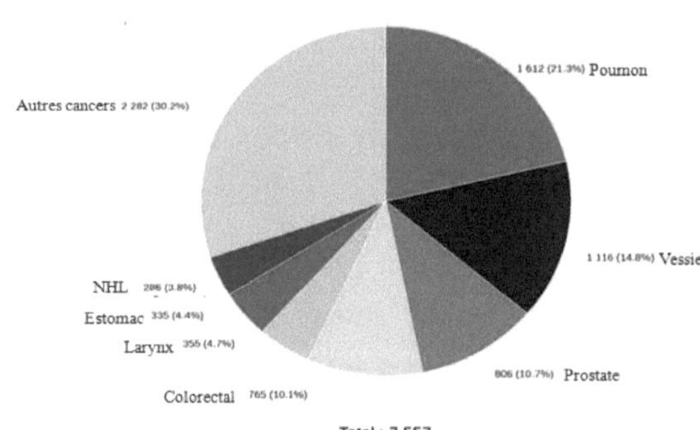

Figure 4: Incidence rates in Tunisia among men over 45 (New Global Cancer Data: GLOBOCAN 2018).

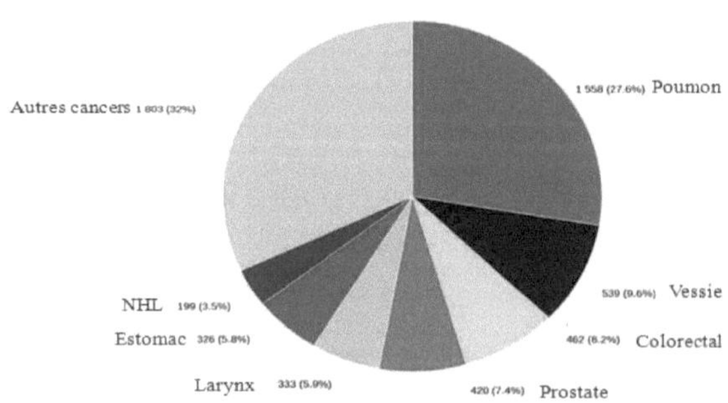

Figure 5: Prostate Cancer mortality rates for Tunisian men over the age of 45 (New Global Cancer Data: GLOBOCAN 2018).

II.2.3. Symptoms

Patients with prostate cancer are asymptomatic in the early stages, as the cancer usually grows slowly and/or may present with symptoms similar to advanced or metastatic BPH. The most revealing signs of prostatic malignancies are urinary disorders such as dysuria, pollakiuria, urinary retention and burning or pain on urination. In addition to these signs, other signs may evoke this pathology such as hematuria, hemospermia, dyserection (Fournier, Valeri et al. 2004, Castillejos-Molina and Gabilondo-Navarro 2016). In advanced stages, prostate cancer patients may experience bone pain in the pelvis, dorsolumbar spine or ribs, hips, upper thighs (Norgaard, Jensen et al. 2010).

II.2.4. Diagnosis

The diagnosis of prostate cancer can be confirmed by several tests:

- **Rectal touch: This** involves palpating the gland with a finger through the rectum, enabling the doctor to detect the size and consistency of the prostate, as well as the presence of any abnormalities detectable by touch (irregularities, hardness of an area, increase in size).

- **Prostate Specific Antigen (PSA) test:** This test has been the second most widely used screening test for prostate cancer since the 1980s. PSA is a protein synthesized by the prostate gland and normally found in small amounts in the bloodstream to liquefy sperm after ejaculation. The concentration of this substance is measured in nanograms per milliliter (ng/ml). Elevation of PSA levels above the usual value (4 ng/ml) indicates the presence of prostate abnormalities, including cancer, benign prostatic hyperplasia or inflammation (prostatitis). The PSA value may temporarily rise following ejaculation or surgery. To date, PSA is the world's leading early diagnostic marker for prostate cancer. The test can also be used to monitor the effectiveness of certain prostate cancer treatments.

- **Prostate biopsies:** This examination is performed using an ultrasound probe and under local anaesthetic. The urologist removes at least 12 fragments of prostate tissue transrectally from different parts of the gland. These biopsies are then examined by the anatomopathologist to confirm the presence of prostate cancer, to specify the aggressiveness of the cancer cells according to the Gleason score, to evaluate the number of positive biopsies, to describe the characteristics of the healthy tissue and to detect the crossing of cancer cells beyond the prostate capsule (Keto and Freedland 2011, Rozet, Hennequin et al. 2016).

II.2.5. Classification and extension

An extension work-up determines the tumor stage, prognosis and therapeutic indications. It is assessed by digital rectal examination (DRE), PSA, prostate biopsies and imaging studies. The TNM classification (Tumor, Node or Ganglion, Metastasis) of prostate cancer is systematically established.

II.2.5.1. PSA

Prostate adenocarcinoma is detected if the PSA level is above the normal serum value of 4 ng/ml, or if there is a successive increase in the PSA value. If the value is between 4 and 10 ng/ml, the free PSA/total PSA ratio would be established. In prostate cancer, the free PSA fraction is lower than in benign prostatic hyperplasia. As a result, this ratio is higher than 20% in BPH and lower than 10% in prostatitis or prostate cancer. In the advanced or metastatic stage, the PSA level is generally greater than or equal to 100 ng/ml (Rozet, Hennequin et al. 2016).

II.2.5.2. Rectal touch

The digital rectal examination (DRE) can help the urologist to assess and classify the disease. A suspicious DRE is associated with an advanced tumor stage and would be a sign to perform prostate biopsies regardless of the PSA value (Rozet, Hennequin et al. 2016).

II.2.5.3. Gleason score

This score, defined by Gleason in 1966, is a grading system in prostate cancer. It is a histopronostic score specifying the degree of glandular differentiation and patterns of cancer infiltration into non-tumoral prostate tissue. The score comprises 5 grades ranging from 1 to 5 (Figure 6). Since adenocarcinoma is often heterogeneous and comprises more than one grade, this score is obtained by adding the two grades in the tumor (from 2 to 10). Observation of a single grade doubles the score, e.g. Gleason score=6 (3+3). Approximately all prostate cancers diagnosed today have a minimum Gleason score of 6, corresponding to a very well-differentiated cancer with a good prognosis. As a result, there is a strong correlation between Gleason score and prognosis (the higher the Gleason score, the more aggressive the cancer and the worse the prognosis). The Gleason score depends on the sum of the majority and minority grades:

- **Grade 3**: The glands are separate and well-formed, varying in size.
- **Grade 4:** Fused or poorly separated glands or infiltrating focus of cribriform masses
- **Grade 5:** Absence of glandular form, infiltrating focus of sheets of independent cells, centered masses of necrosis (comedocarcinoma).

II.2.5.4. ISUP grade

The ISUP (International Society of Urological Pathology) grade resembles the Gleason score, and represents a new, more precise "Grading" system divided into 5 prognostic groups (Table 1) (Rozet, Hennequin et al. 2016).

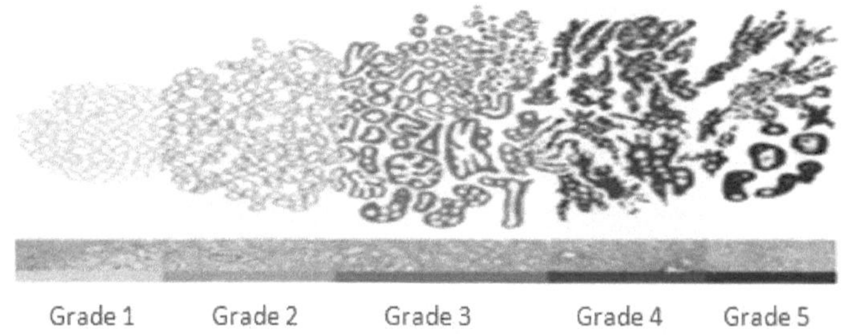

Figure 6: Differentiation of the prostate gland

(https://www.livres-medicaux.com/pathologie-des-voies-urinaires-excretrices.html)

Grades 1 and 2 have very well-separated and shaped glands of the same size and are not included in the grading, Grade 3 has well-separated and shaped glands of different sizes, Grade 4 where the glands are poorly separated or fused, Grade 5 where the glandular shape is absent and the focus is infiltrated by sheets of independent cells.

Table 1: Gleason score and ISUP grade for prostate cancer (Rozet, Hennequin et al. 2016).

Gleason score	ISUP grade
6 (3+3)	Grade 1
7 (3+4)	Grade 2
7 (4+3)	Grade 3
8 (4+4) and 8 (5+3)	Grade 4
9 and 10	Grade 5

II.2.5.5. TNM classification
a. TNM clinical classification (2010)

The TNM classification of prostate cancer defined by the seventh edition of the 2009 classification of malignant tumors is shown in Table 2 (Rozet, Hennequin et al. 2016).

Table 2: TNM classification of prostate cancer (Rozet, Hennequin et al. 2016).

T: Primary tumor	N: Node or lymph node

T0: primary tumor not found
T1: tumor neither palpable on rectal examination nor visible on imaging
   T1a: tumor occupying less than 5% of resected tissue with Gleason score < 7 or absence of grade 4 or 5
   T1b: tumor occupying more than 5% of resected tissue or a Gleason score ≥ 7 or presence of grade 4 or 5
   T1c: tumour discovered on prostate biopsy due to elevated PSA value
T2: tumor confined to the prostate
	Nx: Regional lymph nodes not evaluated
	
	N0: No regional lymph node metastasis
	
	N1: Regional lymph node involvement
	N1mi: lymph node metastasis ≤ 0.2 cm (optional)

T2a: tumour reaching half a lobe or less
   T2b: tumour reaching more than half a lobe but not both lobes
   T2c: tumor reaching both lobes T3: extension beyond the prostate gland
   T3a: uni or bilateral extra-prostatic extension
   T3b: uni- or bilateral extension to the seminal vesicles
T4: tumour attached to or involving structures other than the seminal vesicles (external sphincter, rectum, elevator muscle, etc.).
anus or pelvic wall)
	M: distant metastases
	
	Mx: distant metastases not assessed
	
	M0: no distant metastases
	
	M1: distant metastases
	
	M1a: non-regional lymph node involvement
	
	M1b: bone involvement
	
	M1c: other sites with or without bone involvement

b. Pathological classification (pTNM)

This is a classification after radical prostatectomy (RP) where stage T1 is excluded from this classification:

- pT0: No tumor identified after radical prostatectomy
- pT2: Tumor limited to the prostate (apex and capsule)
    - pT2a: Involvement of half a lobe or less
    - pT2b: Involvement of more than half of one lobe without involvement of the other lobe
    - pT2c: Involvement of both lobes
- pT3: Extension beyond the Capsule
    - T3a: Uni- or bilateral extra-capsular extension including the bladder neck
    - T3b: Extension to seminal vesicles (uni- or bilateral)

- pT4: Extension to adjacent organs (external urethral sphincter, rectum, levator ani muscles, pelvic wall) (Rozet, Hennequin et al. 2016).

c. AMICO classification

Based on the risk of tumor progression, D'Amico proposed a classification of localized malignant tumors to better guide management and give an idea of the percentage of recurrence. This classification is presented in Table 3.

Table 3: D'Amico classification (Rozet, Hennequin et al. 2016)

AMICO classification	
Low risk	PSA< 10 ng/mL + Gleason score ≤ 6 + clinical stage T1c or T2a.
Intermediate risk	PSA between 10 and 20 ng/mL or score Gleason 7 or stage T2b.
High risk	PSA> 20 ng/mL or Gleason score ≥ 8 or clinical stage T2c.

II.2.5.6. Assessment of extension

Extension work-up depends on the D'Amico classification: if the patient is at low risk, the urologist may recommend magnetic resonance imaging (MRI) as an option along with other diagnostic tests. If the patient is at intermediate risk, a prostate and lymph node MRI or pelvic CT scan, bilateral ilio-obturator lymph node curage and bone tomoscintigraphy (if grade 4 predominates) will be recommended. However, if the patient is at high risk, a bone scan, abdominal ultrasound and chest X-ray will be requested by the physician.

II.2.6. Treatment of prostate cancer

II.2.6.1. Treatment options a.

Active surveillance

Patients at low risk of progression according to the D'Amico classification (PSA<10 ng/ml AND Gleason ≤ 6 AND T2a) or Gleason score 6 should have their PSA and prostate biopsies regularly monitored every 6 months. These patients have a life expectancy of over 10 years, since the cancer is unlikely to progress or to progress only slowly. Discontinuation of active surveillance depends on the PSA value doubling in the short term and on the appearance of grade 4 or 5 cancer on prostate biopsies (Rozet, Hennequin et al. 2016).

b.Total prostatectomy

This is a curative treatment offered to patients under 75 with localized or locally advanced cancer and a life expectancy of over 10 years. It involves complete removal of the prostate gland and seminal vesicles, accompanied by vesico-urethral anastomosis. In the case of localized intermediate-risk or high-risk prostate cancer, radical prostatectomy may be combined with bilateral ilioobturator curage, or even extensive pelvic curage. However, surgery presents certain side effects such as Urinary incontinence (10-15%), erectile dysfunction (60-90%), infertility and vesico-urethral anastomosis stenosis (1%) (Rozet, Hennequin et al. 2016).

II.2.6.2. Therapeutic strategies

The choice of treatment depends on age, life expectancy, D'Amico classification and mictional disorders. Some treatments are curative, others palliative:

a. Curative treatments

These treatments are considered for patients with a life expectancy of over 10 years and under 75 years of age. In the case of a low-risk localized cancer, it is legitimate to propose active surveillance to the patient, if not various standard treatments that have been validated, noting radical prostatectomy, interstitial radiotherapy (brachytherapy) and external radiotherapy (76-78 Gy). For intermediate-risk malignant tumors, the treatment options recommended by the oncology committee of the Association Française de l'Urologie (AFU) are radical prostatectomy combined with extensive lymph node dissection, external radiotherapy with a dose greater than 76-78 Gy, and external radiotherapy with short 6-month hormone therapy according to the Bolla protocol. Optionally, brachytherapy in this case can be combined with external radiotherapy. Hormonal radiotherapy and radical prostatectomy with extensive lymph node dissection in a young person are the standard treatments for high-risk prostate cancers (Rozet, Hennequin et al. 2016).

b. Palliative treatments

These treatments are aimed at metastatic patients with a life expectancy of less than 10 years, aged over 75. Surgical (pulpectomy or orchiectomy) or medical (hormone therapy) androgen suppression would be a first-line treatment in the palliative management of locally advanced or metastatic cancers. Since the prostate gland and prostate cancer are linked to the presence of testosterone, androgen suppression with LH-RH agonists or antagonists aims to lower testosterone levels in the body. As a result, testosterone levels are below 0.5 ng/ml during castration. This androgenic suppression can cause early side effects such as hot flushes, loss of libido, erectile dysfunction and asthenia, as well as late side effects such as osteoporosis, muscle loss, depression, neuropsychological disorders and lipid disorders. Hormonal treatment involves :

- The LH-RH agonists used are designed to saturate this signaling pathway, gradually leading to the cessation of testosterone. The drugs used are Decapeptyl® and Zoladex®. These treatments can cause a sudden "Flare-up" in testosteronemia before it collapses, necessitating co-prescription of an anti-androgen for at least a month.

- LH-RH antagonists directly block this pathway to collapse testosteronemia levels without the risk of Flare-up noting Firmagon®.

- Steroidal anti-androgens (Androcur®) or non-steroidal anti-androgens (Casodex®) aimed at direct blockade of the androgen receptor and sometimes at central inhibition of steroidal anti-androgens.

- Traditionally, the urologist prescribes agonist or antagonist monotherapy as a first-line treatment. In high-risk metastatic patients, a complete androgen blockade (BAC) (agonist + anti-androgen or antagonist alone) may then be required. If the PSA value rises after BAC, anti-androgen must be discontinued in this state in order to achieve a drop in PSA, otherwise second-generation hormone therapy (estrogen, estracyt) would be considered. Unfortunately, this hormonosensitivity does not last long (24-36 months), and is referred to as the "castration-resistant phase of prostate cancer" (CRPC). The latter is defined by several criteria according to AFU recommendations (Rozet, Hennequin et al. 2016):

- Testosterone levels (<50 ng/dL or 1.7 nmol/L) ;

- Three PSA increases with an interval of 2 weeks and a value greater than 2 ng/ml;

- Withdrawal of anti-androgen for more than 4 to 6 weeks;

- Clinical (bone pain) or radiological (bone scan or abdomino-pelvic CT) progression.

In minimally symptomatic patients with castration resistance, abiraterone acetate (Zytiga ®) (androgen synthesis inhibitor) and enzalutamide (androgen receptor blocker) can be prescribed as a further step in hormone therapy escalation in prostate cancer patients.

In addition to hormone therapy, chemotherapy is a palliative treatment for symptomatic metastatic prostate cancer resistant to castration. Docetaxel (taxotere®) is the first treatment considered in this case, in combination with prednisone (microtubule inhibitors). For those with a good response to docetaxel, cabazitaxel (Jevtana®) would be prescribed next (Rozet, Hennequin et al. 2016). Nevertheless the adverse effects of biphosphonates (zoledronic acid, Zometa®) on patient health, these molecules can be used as palliative treatment given their ability to inhibit bone resorption linked to osteoclastic activity (Rozet, Hennequin et al. 2016).

II.2.6.3. Monitoring

The disease is monitored for at least ten years. Initially, monitoring is performed every 6 months for the first 5 years, then every year thereafter, depending on the stage and severity of the tumour. The aim of monitoring is to detect recurrence and assess post-treatment complications. This follow-up would be as follows:

↓ Clinical: signs of local or general
extension↓ Biological:

- PSA assay :
  - After radical prostatectomy, PSA levels must be less than 0.2 ng/ml
  - After brachytherapy or radiotherapy, the PSA must be below the nadir PSA (lowest PSA observed after radiotherapy) + 2ng/ml according to the ***Phoenix*** criteria.
  - After other therapeutic modalities, the PSA value must be stable and low.
- Testosteronemia: the testosteronemia value must be less than 0.5 ng/ml if the patient is on hormonal treatment.

➕ Side effects: you should always monitor the side effects of prescribed treatments.

II.2.7. Etiology

Several risk factors may coexist to trigger the development of this pathology.

II.2.7.1. Age

Age is a major factor in the increased risk of prostate cancer. The incidence of this cancer increases with age. Typically, 95% of men diagnosed with prostate cancer are between 57 and 88 years of age. According to worldwide statistics during 2000 and 2008, 1% of patients are aged between 40 and 44 (Leitzmann and Rohrmann 2012).

II.2.7.2. Ethnic origin

The incidence of prostate cancer varies between continents and populations. The risk of developing prostate cancer in men over the age of 45 in relation to the estimated total number of new cases of cancer patients (2018 statistics) is around 35.3% in the European population, 23.3% in the Asian population, 18.4'% in the American population and 6.3% in the African population. However, countries in Oceania have a very low risk of developing prostate cancer (1.8%) (New Global Cancer Data: GLOBOCAN 2018) (Figure 7).

II.2.7.3. Family history
The incidence of developing prostate cancer is two to five times greater if the father or brother is a carrier of this disease (Daniyal, Siddiqui et al. 2014).

II.2.7.4. Environment

People's environment and lifestyle influence the development of prostate cancer. Indeed, diet may influence the development of prostate cancer. Some studies have confirmed that a diet high in animal fat and low in fiber (lycopene) may increase the risk of developing prostate cancer, and vice versa (Alexander, Mink et al. 2010, Leitzmann and Rohrmann 2012).

II.2.7.5. Physical activities

Men with low levels of physical activity are more likely to develop prostate cancer (Giovannucci, Liu et al. 2005, Antonelli, Freedland et al. 2009).

II.2.7.6. Chemical exposure

Science has confirmed the effect of certain pesticides in increasing the risk of prostate cancer (Parent, Désy et al. 2009).

II.2.7.7. Hormones

High levels of testosterone and estrogen in the human body may increase the incidence of prostate cancer (Michaud, Daugherty et al. 2006, Yao, Till et al. 2011).

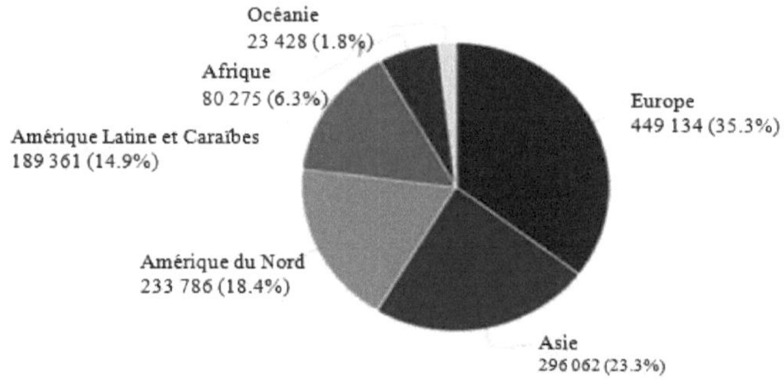

Figure 7: Prostate cancer incidence rates by continent

(New Global Cancer Data: GLOBOCAN 2018)

II.2.7.8. Sexual activity and sexually transmitted diseases

Infection with *Trichomonas vaginalis* (human parasite) is associated with the risk of developing prostate cancer, according to various studies (Sutcliffe , Giovannucci et al. 2006, Stark, Judson et al. 2009). However, it has been shown that Gonorrhea infection (a sexually transmitted infection) may be associated with prostate cancer in Latin men living in the USA (Cheng, Witte et al. 2010). In addition, it has been suggested that excessive sexual activity may increase the risk of developing prostate cancer for a number of reasons, such as increased testosterone levels and changing partners, making sexual diseases more easily transmitted (Leitzmann and Rohrmann 2012). Conversely, ejaculation frequency is inversely correlated with increased risk of this disease (Leitzmann, Platz et al. 2004).

II.2.7.9. Other factors

Other factors are associated with the development of prostate cancer, such as obesity, excessive calcium intake and the presence of chronic inflammation or prostatic intraepithelial neoplasia (PIN) (Murata, Takayama et al. 2012) in young people before the age of 50 (Hirata, Hinoda et al. 2007, Leitzmann and Rohrmann 2012).

II.2.7.10. Genetic factor

Individual susceptibility to xenobiotics (drugs, pollutants, foods), to which each person is necessarily exposed, depends on the expression of xenobiotic metabolism enzymes. This expression varies between individuals according to physiopathological, environmental and genetic factors. In addition, various genome-wide association studies (GWAS) (Nakagawa, Akamatsu et al. 2016, Benafif, Kote-Jarai et al. 2018) have emphasized the importance of genetic polymorphism of the genes involved, in other metabolic pathways such as folate metabolism pathways (Collin, Metcalfe et al. 2009), immune function (Michaud, Daugherty et al. 2006), xenobiotic metabolism pathways (Murata, Watanabe et al. 2001), oxidative stress response (Choi, Neuhouser et al. 2008) and DNA repair (Rybicki, Conti et al. 2004, Hirata, Hinoda et al. 2007) in the onset of prostate cancer.

B. Somatic changes in prostate cancer

I. Genetic alterations

In addition to genetic predisposition factors, somatic genetic and epigenetic alterations in certain genes are recurrently associated with the development and/or progression of prostate cancer. To date, the identification of certain genes that alter prostate cancer has been established. These include :

- RNaseL (HPC1, lq22), MSR1 (8p), ELAC2/HPC2 (17p11) in hereditary CP (Schoenborn, Nelson et al. 2013)

- PTEN, BRCA2, TP53, FOXP1, RYOP, MAGI, RB1, SPOP, SPINK1, ADAMTS-1
  etc. in localized tumors (Schoenborn, Nelson et al. 2013).
  - ADAMTS-1 is a gene encoding an ADAMTS protein family consisting of a disintegrin and a metalloproteinase with a thrombospondin type 1 motif. This gene is responsible for fertility, growth, organ morphology and development (Shindo, Kurihara et al. 2000). In prostate cancer, this gene is poorly elucidated, but is probably involved in the early stage of prostate cancer development, playing an anti-angiogenic role (Gustavsson, Wang et al. 2009).

- **Genes that interact with androgen receptors (ARs):** ASXL2, NKX3-1, FOXA1, TOP2B and are altered in advanced stages: metastasis and resistance to hormone therapy (Schoenborn, Nelson et al. 2013).

- **Transcription factor genes:** FOXA, FOXO which are involved in advanced stages (metastasis and resistance to hormone therapy) (Schoenborn, Nelson et al. 2013).

- FOXO4 is a subclass O gene of the Forkhead family of transcription factors. When displaced to the nucleus, this gene promotes transcription of downstream FOXO targets. FOXO4 regulates several cellular pathways such as apoptosis, longevity, oxidative stress, insulin signaling and cell cycle progression (Obsil and Obsilova 2008). This gene is implicated in advanced stage and hormone therapy resistance in prostate cancer (Huang, Li et al. 2018).

Oncogenes and tumor suppressor genes: PTEN, TP53, RB1, KRAS, BRAF, PDCD4 (Schoenborn, Nelson et al. 2013).

- PDCD4 is a programmed cell death gene. It is located in the nucleus and promotes apoptosis. This gene is modulated by cytokines. Recently, it has been confirmed that this gene plays a major role in advanced metastatic and hormone therapy-resistant prostate cancer (Zennami, Choi et al. 2019).

Chromatin remodeling genes: CHD1, CHD5, MLL2 in metastatic and hormone therapy-resistant stages (Schoenborn, Nelson et al. 2013).

Genes involved in the cell cycle: PI3KCA, PTEN, mTOR, CDKN1B, MED12 (Schoenborn, Nelson et al. 2013).

In addition to genetic alterations, epigenetic alterations can also modulate inter-individual variability in gene expression. Hence, epigenetic regulation is defined as a set of mechanisms that can act on cellular phenotypes, leading to a change in activity or function without involving DNA sequence modifications, and that are heritable during mitosis or meiosis (Heard and Martienssen 2014). The main epigenetic mechanisms are posttranslational histone modifications, histone variants, DNA methylation, non-coding RNAs and ATP-dependent chromatin remodeling complexes (Kyburz, Karouzakis et al. 2014) (Figure 8).

⬥ **Epithelial-mesenchymal transition genes:** Epithelial-mesenchymal transition (EMT) is a process by which epithelial cells undergo transformation into mesenchymal cells. This process is involved in various pathological phenomena, such as tumor progression and fibrosis. It is characterized by loss of cell-cell adhesion, degradation of the basal lamina and acquisition of migratory and invasive capacities. EMT has been associated with metastatic dissemination and poor prognosis in certain cancers(Roche, 2018). Research has highlighted the role of different transcription factors in the induction of EMT, as well as the reversibility of this process, exemplified by mesenchymal-epithelial transition (MET). Understanding EMT is important in the context of research into cancer and other diseases, as it could lead to the development of new therapeutic strategies (Ribatti, Tamma, & Annese, 2020). Among the EMT genes is Zeb-1, which is involved in the progression, invasion, migration and metastasis of various types of cancer, including breast, lung, pancreatic, colon, uterine and others. Zeb-1 has been shown to regulate the expression of genes associated with tumor progression, invasion and metastasis. Its overexpression is associated with poor clinical outcome in cancer patients, making it a potential biomarker of poor prognosis. Zeb-1 acts by promoting epithelial-mesenchymal transition. It has also been suggested that Zeb-1 confers plasticity to breast cancer cells by conferring stem cell characteristics. Thus, Zeb-1 plays an important role in tumor progression and cancer cell plasticity, making it a potential target for the development of cancer therapies (Madany, Thomas, & Edwards, 2018; Perez-Oquendo & Gibbons, 2022; Zhang, Xu, Li, & Han, 2019).

II. Epigenetic mechanisms and factors associated with the development of prostate cancer

II.1. Histone acetylation and DNA methylation

DNA methylation is an important mechanism in the epigenetic regulation of gene expression. Indeed, it is considered a key element in the formation and maintenance of chromatin structure, gene regulation and other fundamental processes. It is a post-replicative modification involving the addition of a methyl CH3 group to the pyrimidine base of cytosine at CpG islands. These are located mainly either near the transcription initiation site, or at the promoter regions of genes (Moore, Le et al. 2013). This methylation is catalyzed by DNA methyltransferases (DNMTs) (Jin, Li et al. 2011, Moore, Le et al. 2013). Whole epigenome association studies (EWAS) have highlighted the association between DNA methylation levels and prostate cancer development and progression. Indeed, hypermethylation at the promoters of HOX family genes and the GSTP1 gene would induce protein underexpression of its targets. In addition, methylation of certain candidate genes could act as biomarkers in prostate cancer. In this context, researchers are proposing to stratify CP stages according to the level of methylation of certain candidate genes despite its difficulty on a clinical scale (Graff, Herman et al. 1995, Cairns, Esteller et al. 2001, Yegnasubramanian, Kowalski et al. 2004, Zhao, Olkhov-Mitsel et al. 2018).

Other than DNA methylation, histone acetylation is a reversible epigenetic mechanism involving the addition of a chemical acetyl group (COCH3) to a positively charged amino acid (Arginine R or Lysine K). The addition of this group generally neutralizes the amino acids, causing an electrostatic change between the negatively-charged DNA and the histones.

This opens up the chromatin structure and increases the accessibility of DNA for transcription (Abbas and Gupta 2008). The main enzymes are histone acetyltransferases (HATs) and histone deacetylases (HDACs). Various studies have examined the effect of these enzymes on the development and/or prognosis of prostate cancer, noting that HDAC1 and HDAC2 are positively associated with Gleason score (Ngollo, Dagdemir et al. 2014).

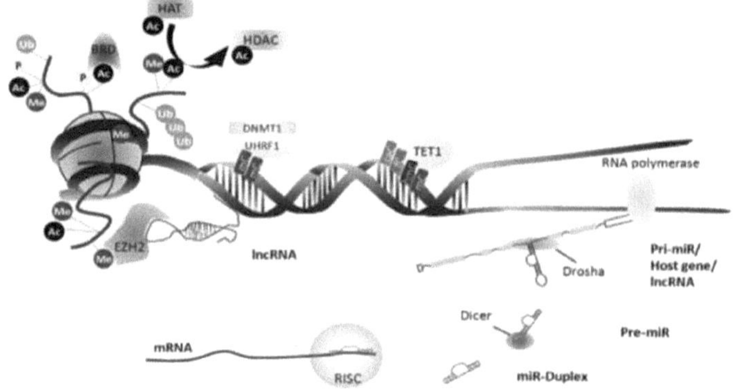

Figure 8: *Epigenetic regulatory mechanisms*

(Kyburz, Karouzakis et al. 2014).

Different mechanisms of epigenetic regulation: DNA methylation, Histone deacetylation, MicroRNA interference. BRD: Barbu complex, HAT: histone acetyl transferases, HDAC: histone deacetylases, Dnmt1: DNA methyltransferase 1, UHRF1: Ubiquitin as with PHD and Ring Finger Domains 1, Ezh2: Skin homolog enhancer 2, LncRNA: long non Coding RNA, TET1: methylcytosine dioxygenase 1, RISC: RNA-induced silencing complex.

II.2.1. Definition of miRs

miRs are small molecules (around 18 to 25 nucleotides) belonging to the non-coding RNA (ncRNA) family. More than 4076 miRs have been identified to date (Bartels and Tsongalis 2009, Chou, Shrestha et al. 2018). These small molecules act in the post-transcriptional regulation of gene expression by binding to the 3'UTR (Untranslated Region) of their target messenger RNAs (mRNAs). Complete or incomplete binding to the target could cause translational repression or also mRNA degradation (Chou, Shrestha et al. 2018).

These small sequences play a very important role in the human organism noting development, apoptosis, growth, metabolism, cell differentiation, proliferation and aging (Lai 2002, Mohr and Mott 2015). Scientific studies have shown that post-transcriptional regulation by miRs affects over 60% of protein-coding genes. As a result, numerous studies have elucidated the association of many diseases with miRs deregulation such as autoimmune inflammatory diseases, endocrine disorders as well as cancer (Bartels and Tsongalis 2009). These miRs can also serve as biomarkers for diagnosis, prognosis and therapy.

II.2.2. Biogenesis of miRs

The biogenesis of mature miRs takes place in four biological process steps (Morgan and Bale 2012):

- ⚓ **Transcription:** This stage takes place in the nucleus, generally by RNA polymerase II, and involves the transcription of miR genes into primary transcripts known as "pri-miRs". These have a 5' cap and a 3' polyadenylated tail, and are very large in size (500 to 3,000 bases) (Figure 9).

- **Cleavage of pri-miR into pre-miR precursor:** The primary transcript is cleaved by the "microprocessor" nuclear protein complex, formed by an RNAase III "Drosha" and a single-stranded RNA-binding protein "DGCR8" (DiGeorge syndrome Critical Region 8). The synthesized pre-miR consists of around 70 nucleotides. Pri-miR splicing could also be another mechanism of pre-miR synthesis independently of the "Drosha-DGCR8" complex.

- **Export to the cytoplasm:** Pre-miR is released into the cytoplasm via protein complexes incorporated into the nuclear membrane, known as Exportin 5 (XPO5). The cooperative binding of pre-miR to the Ran-GTP cofactor forms a double-stranded RNA structure of over 14 bp, enabling XPO5 to export pre-miR outside the nucleus by hydrolyzing GTP.

- **Cleavage into miR**: The release of pre-miR into the cytoplasm in its stem-loop form is followed by its cleavage by a "TRBP" (TaR Binding Protein) endonuclease of the DRBP (dsRNA Binding Protein) family and a cytoplasmic "RNAseIII" endonuclease, forming a mature, double-stranded miR. Elimination of the loop structure is achieved by the "Dicer-TRBP" complex, separating the two strands of the stem and attaching one of them to the "RISC" complex (RNA-Induced Silencing Complex), thus inducing the formation of the miRISC complex, which is mediated by the presence of AGO family proteins (1-4). Finally, the "mature miR" guide strand remains bound to the RISC protein for subsequent binding to its target mRNA. The "miR passenger" strand, on the other hand, separates from the duplex and degrades.

Aberrant expression of miRs could affect several biological processes in cancers such as apoptosis, invasion, drug resistance and tumor proliferation and metastasis (Iorio and Croce 2012). Various miRs have been deregulated in prostate cancer lines (DU145, LnCaP and PC3), as well as in patient cancer cells (Vanacore, Boccellino et al. 2017). Two types of miRs are mentioned:

- **OncomiRs overexpressed in prostate cancer:** miR-141, miR-20a, miR-21, miR-195, miR-375, miR-221/miR-222, miR-141, miR-375, miR-18a, miR-4534, miR-650, miR-32, miR-106/miR-25, miR-125b etc.

- **tumor suppressor miRs that are underexpressed in prostate cells:** miRs: miR-34a, miR-143/145, miR-205, miR-488 , miR-34a, miR-145, miR-224, miR-452, miR-200b, miR-382, miR-372, miR-17-92a, miR-27a, miR-135-a-1, miR-204-5p, miR-30a, let-7, miR-133/miR-146a etc .

However, since the discovery of miRs in 1993, various studies have emphasized the usefulness of these small molecules in the diagnosis of prostate cancer as diagnostic biomarkers. In addition, a panel of miRs identified for prostate cancer diagnosis could be used alongside PSA in the early diagnosis of patients. On the other hand, certain miRs have been identified as biomarkers of prostate cancer tumor progression and biochemical recurrence after radical prostatectomy.

- **Hsa-miR-101-1: This is** a microRNA-containing precursor that has been found to significantly decrease in LT and Ar compared to IBA in various brain regions. MicroRNA-101 (miR-101) is an RNA gene affiliated to the miRNA class and is associated with several diseases, including lung and breast cancer. miR-101 targets the proteasome maturation protein POMP, resulting in altered proteasome assembly and activity, which inhibits cell growth and induces apoptosis. Furthermore, miR-101-1 has been shown to inhibit nasopharyngeal carcinoma cell proliferation and cisplatin resistance by down-regulating ZIC5 targeting. The human microRNA precursor hsa-mir-101 (hsa-mir-101-1) is involved in various biological processes and has been studied in different contexts, such as brain regions and cancer cells (C. Wang et al., 2014; C. Z. Wang et al., 2018).

- **Hsa-mir-96-5p**: Hsa-mir-96-5p is located on exon 1 of chromosome 7q32.2 and plays both an oncomir and tumor suppressor role, depending on the type of cancer. In pancreatic cancer, miR-96-5p appears to be involved in tumor suppressor function by suppressing KRAS activity, whereas in prostate cancer it appears as a metastamiR or oncomiR. Various studies demonstrate that the miR-183-96-182 cluster plays an important role in oncogenesis, cancer progression, tumor invasion and metastasis. The prostate tumor suppressor gene PTEN has been shown to be regulated by miR-183-5p and miR-96-5p and to promote cell proliferation in breast cancer by directly affecting the tumor suppressor gene FOXO3a and the cyclin-dependent kinase inhibitors p27Kip1 and p21Cip1. Thus, the miR-183-96-182 cluster is a prospective biomarker candidate for prognosis of prostate cancer. In addition, miR-96-5p down-regulates the tumor suppressor FOXO1, which induces cell cycle arrest and cell death in endometrial cancer. In addition, FOXO1 acts as a repressor of androgen receptor activity, which is the central oncogenic pathway in the development of prostate cancer. There is a study showing that prostate cancer metastasis is promoted by stimulation of the TGF-β and SMAD genes by inducing miR-96-5p and activating the mTOR pathway. Another study shows that miR-96 can promote bone metastasis and contribute to reduced survival rates. This study argues that miR-96-5p could be used as a prognostic marker and potential target of therapies for metastatic prostate cancer. (H. Wang, Ma, Li, & Wang,

2020).

- **Hsa-miR-548ac:** Located on exon 1 of chromosome 1p13.1. Previous investigations have shown that miR-548ac has 69 genes located in almost all chromosomes. Some investigations have also shown that miR-548ac may be involved in different types of cancer, including prostate cancer, breast cancer and pancreatic cancer. It may play the role of oncogene or tumor suppressor, depending on the type of cancer. In pancreatic cancer, overexpression of miR-548ac suppressed cell migration, proliferation and invasion, while its silencing restored cancer migration, proliferation and invasion (Sharma & Gupta, 2020). In prostate cancer, this miR acts as an oncogene. Several studies have shown that there is a difference in miR-548ac expression in tumor and normal tissues, and overexpression of miR-548ac is observed in prostate tumor tissues. Upregulation of miR-548ac expression was significantly correlated with high-risk Gleason scores. One study suggests that miR-548ac represses the expression of PTEN, which plays a key role in regulating the PI3k / AKT pathway, the most important signalling pathway regulating cellular processes such as cell cycle, survival, metabolism, motility, genomic instability and angiogenesis, and frequent changes in prostate cancer. (Sharma & Gupta, 2020).

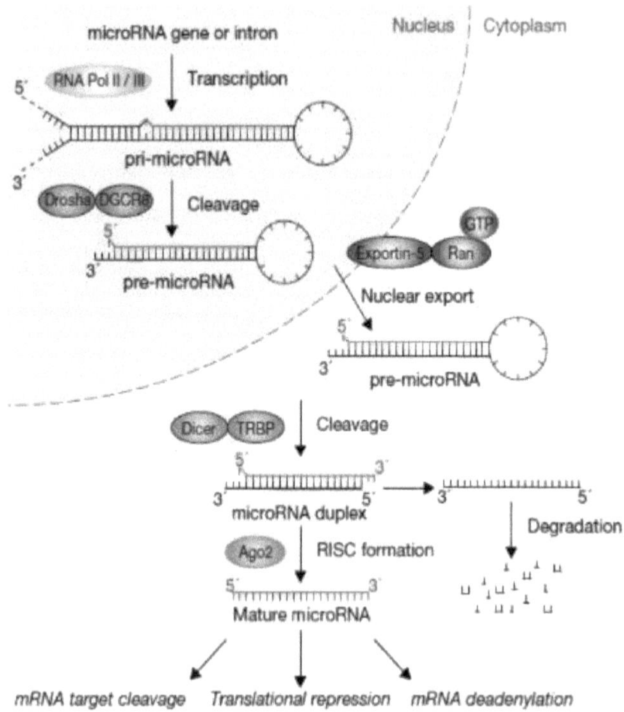

Figure 9: Main steps in microRNA biogenesis (Srikok, Chuammitri et al. 2016).

Nucleus: Nucleus , Cytoplasm:Cytoplasm, microRNA gene or intron: microRNA genes or introns, RNA Pol II/III: RNA polymerase II/III, pri-microRNA: pri-microRNA, Cleavage:Clivage,pre-microRNA: pre-microRNA, Nuclear export: Export Nucléaire ,microRNA duplex: Duplex microRNA, RISC formation, Mature microRNA, mRNA Target cleavage, Translational repression, mRNA deadenylation.

Objective

Our main objective in this study is to deepen our understanding of prostate cancer, a complex disease resulting from the interaction of various environmental, genetic and hormonal factors, as well as somatic alterations in prostate cells. Being the third most common form of cancer among men in Tunisia, this disease has been relatively unexplored in local scientific research.

With this in mind, our study focuses specifically on the genetic and epigenetic aspects of prostate cancer. The ultimate goal is to analyze the expression level of the Zeb-1 gene and its targets, namely Hsa-miR-548ac, Hsa-miR-96-5p and Hsa-miR-101-1. We aim to establish significant correlations between these gene expressions and the epidemiological and anatomopathological data of prostate cancer patients.

In short, our approach aims to enrich our knowledge of this disease by exploring epigenetic aspects, thus paving the way for new perspectives in the understanding, diagnosis and treatment of prostate cancer in Tunisia.

Materials & Methods

Study population

This is a prospective study of 14 prostate cancer patients with a mean age of 72.66 and two healthy subjects aged 68.99 ± 8.51 recruited from the Urology Department of Charles Nicolle Hospital, Tunis. This work was carried out on fresh tumor sections and healthy tissue which were preserved at -20°C in tubes containing RPMI (Roswell Park Memorial Institute medium) in order to maintain tissue integrity. The epidemiological and/or clinical characteristics of the study population will be detailed in the following paragraphs.

I.1.   Epidemiological and clinico-pathological data on the study population

Clinical and anatomopathological data were collected from the records of patients hospitalized in the Urology Department of Charles Nicolle Hospital, Tunis (Table 4). This work was approved by the Ethics Committee of Charles Nicolle Hospital, Tunis. All participants gave their informed and signed consent.

Table 4: Clinical, anatomopathological and epidemiological characteristics of prostate cancer patients

Clinical and epidemiological data and Anatomopathology	Number of CP patients (n=14)
Gender	Men
Average age	72 .67
Average PSA (ng/ml)	148.93
Gleason score Gleason score <6 Gleason score = 6-7 Gleason score >7	 4 (33.33%) 5 (33.33%) 5 (33.33%)
Progression of metastasis M_0 M_+ Lack of information	 5(33.33%) 09 (66.67%) 0
Tumor recurrence Yes No Lack of information	 0 0 14(100%)
Target treatment Palliative Curative Lack of information	 5(40%) 9(60%) 0
Smoking Yes No Lack of information	 09(66.67%) 5(33.33%) 0
Number of packs/year < 20 PY ≥ 20 PY No information	 2(13.33%) 7(53.33%) 5(33.33%)
Alcohol consumption Yes No Lack of information	 4(26.66%) 09(66.67%) 1(6.66%)

Occupational exposure	
Yes	1(6.66%)
No	6(46.66%)
Lack of information	7(46.66%)
HTA (Hypertension)	
Yes	5(40%)
No	9(60%)

I.2. Hardware
Solutions, buffers and kits

- Trizol(Ivitrogen)

- Chloroform

- Isopropanol

- Ethanol(75%,100%)

- Sodium acetate

- RNase Free Water

- dNTP(100mM)

- Taq buffer(10X)

- Mgcl^2(25mM)

- oligo(dt)12-18(500ug/ml)

- Retrotranscription kit: MMLV Reverse Transcriptase Kit(REF :28025-013)

- Retrotranscription kit for microRNA: go Taq ® G2 Flexi DNA Polymerase (Reference:M7805)

- qPCR Kit: 5X HOT FIREPol® EvaGreen® qPCR Supermix(REF: EP2501716)

- Sequences of primers used: The primers used are described in Table 5:

Table 5: Sequences of primers used for Zeb-1 and the 3 miRs

Gene/ miRs	Primer sequences (5' -> 3')
Zeb-1	**F:** AGGATGACAGAAAGGAAGGGCA **R:** TGCATCTGACTCGCATTCATCA
miR-548ac	**F:** GGACGGTAGCAAGCAAAGAGTGTGCTACTAGGTTA **R:** GGGATTCTGGAAGATGATGATGACGTATTAGGTTG
miR-101-1	**F:** GGACGGTAGCAAGCAAAGAGTGTGTGCCATCCTTC **R:** GGGATTCTGGAAGATGATGATGACTGCCCTGGCTC
miR-96-5p	**F:** GGACGGTAGCAAGCAAAGAGTGTGTTTCCCATATT **R:** GGGATTCTGGAAGATGATGATGACTGGCCGATTTT

II.   Methods
II.1.   Nucleic acid extraction (genomic DNA and total RNA) from fresh tumour tissue

The classic Trizol triple extraction method enables simultaneous isolation of RNA, DNA and proteins from the same cell or tissue sample. This method is based on the use of a solution of guanidium isothiocyanate and phenol (Trizol), enabling lysis of the cell and dissociation of nucleoprotein complexes, while maintaining the integrity of the nucleic acids. These molecules are then separated into isolated fractions, which are subsequently recovered by sequential precipitation. Nucleic acid extraction is carried out in the following stages:

3/1/1. Tissue homogenization and molecule separation (DNA, RNA)

The frozen tissue is first ground with a mortar and pestled in liquid nitrogen until it reduces to a powder. Then 1ml of TRIzol is added (for a weight of 50 à 100 mg of tissue) to homogenize it. The resulting homogenate is transferred to an

Eppendorf tube and incubated for 5 min at room temperature. Next, 200ul chloroform is added, followed by vigorous inversion shaking, then reincubated for 2-3 min at room temperature. The resulting mixture is then centrifuged (12,000 g: 15 min: 4°C). This separates the solution into three phases: an aqueous phase containing RNA, an interphase containing DNA and proteins, and an organic phase.

II.1.2. Selective isolation of total RNA

To extract the RNA, the aqueous phase (upper phase) is collected in a new tube, to which 200 µL of isopropanol is added to precipitate the RNA, followed by incubation at room temperature for 10 min and centrifugation (12,000g : 151 : 4°C). The RNA pellet is then washed with 1 ml of 75% ethanol, vortexed briefly and centrifuged (7500g : 5 min ;4°c) to remove all traces of salt precipitate. The resulting pellet is oven-dried at 37°C for 10 min and suspended in 50 µL RNase-free water. To re-precipitate the RNA, 10 µL of 3M sodium acetate and 2V of pure ethanol are added, and the mixture is left to precipitate at -20°C for 30 min, followed by centrifugation (12,000g: 15 min: 4°C). To remove all traces of ethanol and facilitate suspension in water, the RNA pellet is dried briefly in an oven at 37°C, then suspended in 30 µL of RNase-Free water by pipetting. The RNA is then stored at -20°C II.

II.2. Evaluation of nucleic acid concentration and purity

Optical density (OD) is measured by spectrophotometer or Nanodrop. The quantity of nucleic acids is estimated by measuring OD at 260 nm, the wavelength at which nucleic acids ensure maximum absorbance in the ultraviolet. One unit of OD corresponds to 50µg/µL of double-stranded DNA and 40µg/µL of RNA. A second OD reading at 280 nm and 230 nm, followed by calculation of the OD260nm/DO280nm and OD260nm/DO230nm ratios, enables nucleic acid purity to be assessed, and any protein or organic contamination to be detected, respectively, with :

- Pure DNA: ratio 260/280 ~ 1.8-2

 - Pure RNA: ratio 260 /280 ~ 2-2.2

- Pure nucleic acid: ratio 260/230 = 2.2

II.3. Study of Zeb-1 gene expression and potential miRs (miR-548ac, miR-101-1, miR-96-5p) by RT-qPCR (relative quantification method)

II.3.1. Analysis of the specificity of primers designated for expression analysis by conventional PCR

In order to validate the specificity of the designated primers to be used in the real-time PCR amplification reaction of the genes of interest (Zeb-1, miR-548ac, miR-101-1, miR-96-5p, GAPDH), a conventional PCR step was first performed on the cDNA. The cDNA is obtained by reverse transcription from the extracted total RNA.

II.3.2. Reverse transcription from total RNA

This reaction involves using a strand of template RNA to synthesize a complementary strand of single-stranded DNA (cDNA), by reverse transcriptase (retrotranscriptase), an enzyme with RNA-dependent DNA polymerase activity. This synthesis takes place in the $5' \rightarrow 3'$ direction, respecting the rules of antiparallelism and complementarity.

In this work, RT was performed on total RNA using the Moleney Murine Leukemia Virus (M-MLV) enzyme and oligo (dT) primers for total cDNA synthesis. The reverse transcription reaction was performed in a final volume of 20 µL. The first step consists of adding 1 ug of total RNA in the presence of 0.5ug dT oligo, 0.83mM dNTP and bi-distilled water (EBD).

The mixture is then incubated at 65°C for 5 min, to denature the secondary structure of the RNA and facilitate primer accessibility. The tube is quickly placed on ice, followed by centrifugation to collect the contents. In a second step, reagents consisting of 2 ul DTT, 1 ul First strand buffer and 1 ul RNAase out are added to the resulting mixture.

The mixture is then incubated at 37°C for 2 min. A volume of 1µL of M-MLV (200 units) is added to the product and incubated at 37°C for 50 min, which corresponds to the temperature of optimal enzyme activity. This step corresponds to cDNA synthesis. Inactivation of the enzyme follows incubation for 15 minutes at 70°C. The total cDNA obtained can be stored at +4°C or -20°C.

II.3.3. Real-time quantitative PCR

The principle of this technique is the same as that of conventional PCR, with real-time monitoring of amplification product accumulation, by detecting the fluorescence emitted at each cycle. This is achieved by inserting a fluorescent intercalating agent (Sybr Green I) that binds non-specifically to the neo-synthesized double-stranded DNA. The fluorescence emitted by this fluorochrome is measured at the end of the elongation phase for each cycle. Fluorescence intensity is directly proportional to the amount of amplification product present.

The amplification curve is used to determine the Ct value, which provides an estimate of the quantity of cDNA initially present. The Ct (Threshold Cycle) corresponds to the amplification cycle where the fluorescence signal is significantly higher than the background noise, and appears at the start of the exponential phase. DNA quantification therefore takes place in the exponential phase, which explains the precision and reproducibility of this technique. Ct is inversely proportional to the amount of starting cDNA (i.e. RNA). The higher the concentration of the starting target molecule in the sample, the fewer the number of cycles required for the fluorescence signal to exceed the detection threshold, and the lower the Ct value. The amplification curve represents the fluorescence values collected at each amplification cycle. If we follow the fluorescence over time, we observe three phases:

+ **Background phase:** The quantity of amplicons produced is insufficient to generate a signal that exceeds the background noise.

+ **Exponential phase:** The quantity of amplification products generates a fluorescence signal above the detection threshold. The number of amplified products doubles with each cycle.

+ **Plateau phase:** Some components become limiting, amplification is no longer exponential.

The specificity of this amplification system is moderately low, given that it is based exclusively on primer pairing, hence the possibility of the formation of aspecific products. A post-PCR melting curve is required to assess the specificity of each product formed. This is achieved by exposing the amplicons to a stepwise increase in temperature, while measuring fluorescence intensity. A drop in fluorescence is observed from the (dissociation temperature) at which 50% of the double-stranded DNA is dissociated (denatured).

qPCR was performed in a final volume of 10µL using 2.5µL of cDNA, in the presence of 2µL of Master mix, 1µL of primers (F and R) and 4.5µL of RNAse free water (RFW) (Table 6).

Table 6: qPCR reaction medium

Reagents	Initial concentration	Final concentration	Volume drawn
Master Mix	5x	2.5x	2µL
Reverse and sense primers	10mM	0.5mM	1µL
cDNA	1000ng/µL	2500ng/µL	2.5µL
RFW	-	-	4.5µL

Quantification was carried out on the Applied Biosystems StepOne real-time PCR system using the following program: initial denaturation for 10 min at 95°C, followed by 45 cycles: 15sec at 95°C (denaturation) and 1 min at 60°C (extension-coupled primer hybridization). At the end of the PCR reaction, a melting curve is run from 60 to 95°C in 0.1°C steps at 0.3% heating rate, to check that only one PCR product has been amplified. If the curve is polymodal, the results should be interpreted with caution, or the experiment repeated with other, more specific primers. If the curve is unimodal, calculation of the primary derivative gives a bell-shaped curve with the abscissa of the maximum being the Tm of the PCR product (amplicon). Determination of the relative expression level of the genes of interest Zeb-1, miR-548ac, miR-101-1, miR-96-5p is carried out using the relative 2 method$^{-\Delta\Delta CT.}$ This method involves firstly calculating the mean Ct of the duplicates obtained for the target gene *as well as that of the reference gene in patients and non-tumor controls. Next, the ΔCT is calculated,* corresponding to the expression of the gene of interest normalized by that of the endogenous gene (GAPDH) such that *ΔCT*= CT $_{target\ gene}$ -CT$_{gène\ reference}$ *also in patients and healthy controls. This is followed by a second normalization to the healthy (non-tumoral) control. Such as:* $\Delta\Delta CT=\Delta CT$ $_{sample}$ - mean ΔCT $_{control,}$ following averaging of *ΔCT* in all healthy controls. Finally, the *relative* expression of *the* target gene is determined by calculating the fold change (FC) using the formula $2^{-\Delta\Delta CT}$. If the FC is less than 0.5, the gene in question is under-expressed in patients compared with non-tumoral controls, whereas if the FC is greater than 2, the target gene is over-expressed. In the absence of deregulation, the FC of the gene amplified in tumor subjects corresponds to a value between 0.5 and 2. For each sample, amplification of the target genes (Zeb-1, miR-548ac, miR-101-1, miR-96-5p) and GAPDH was performed in triplicate.

III. **Bioinformatics analysis :**

An in silico analysis was performed to identify microRNAs that could target Zeb-

1 mRNA using bioinformatics tools available online. In our study, we identified the Zeb-1 marker as a potential target for miR-548ac, miR-101-1 and miR-96-5p using miRmap (www.mirmap.ezlab.org) and Target Scan (www.targetscan.org).

IV. Statistical tests :

In the context of our research, data analysis was carried out using SPSS software, version 24.0. The results obtained were interpreted using a battery of relevant statistical tests. The Kruskal-Wallis test, a non-parametric test, was used to examine variations between several unpaired groups, based on the comparison of medians. In contrast, Student's t-test, a parametric test, was used to assess differences between two independent groups, focusing on the comparison of means. Relationships between different quantitative variables were explored via the Pearson correlation test, a parametric test for assessing the strength and direction of linear relationships. The results of these analyses were graphically represented using box-plots. It should be noted that the significant error threshold was maintained at 0.05 ($\alpha = 0.05$) to ensure the statistical robustness of the conclusions drawn from this study.

Results

In addition to risk factors of genetic and environmental origin, somatic genetic and epigenetic alterations in certain genes are recurrently associated with the development or progression of prostate cancer. Thus, in this book, we are interested in characterizing somatic alterations in association with prostate cancer diagnosis and/or prognosis, while focusing on microRNAs. miRs are small molecules (around 18 to 25 nucleotides) belonging to the non-coding RNA family. These small molecules act in the post-transcriptional regulation of gene expression by binding to the 3'UTR region of their target messenger RNA. Complete or incomplete binding to the target may cause translational repression or mRNA degradation. In humans, miRs play an important role in the regulation of development, apoptosis, growth, differentiation and cell proliferation.

In this work, we studied the expression profile of the Zeb-1 gene and these three target miRs to understand the mechanism of action between them.

I.   Control of primer pair specificity by conventional PCR
In the present work, the first step following nucleic acid extraction and reverse transcription of total RNA was to check the specificity of the primers designated for qPCR. This was done using a conventional PCR reaction based on cDNA. Agarose gel electrophoretic analysis of the PCR products revealed the presence of amplification bands of the expected size, corresponding to the cDNAs of the genes of interest. This indicates, firstly, the presence of good-quality cDNA that can be used for a subsequent reaction and, secondly, the specificity of the primers designed for qPCR.

II.   Development of the qPCR technique

The aim of this section was to analyze the expression levels of the Zeb-1, miR-548ac, miR-101-1 and miR-96-5p genes in patients compared with non-tumor controls, using real-time PCR. The amplification curve shown below illustrates the number of PCR cycles on the abscissa, and the fluorescence emitted (on a logarithmic scale) on the ordinate. This curve reflects the amount of cDNA present in the reaction medium at each amplification cycle. The Ct value is determined by projecting the point of intersection between the fluorescence curve and the gene-specific detection threshold onto the x-axis (Figure 10).

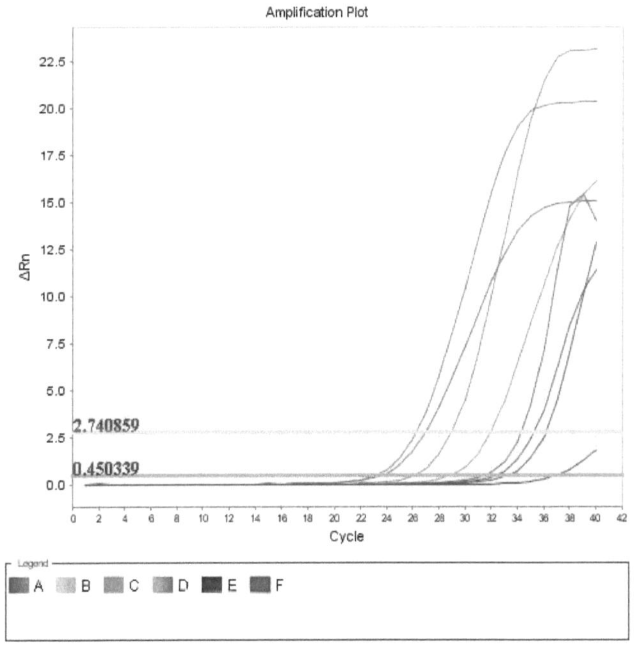

Figure 10: Amplification curve for Zeb-1, GAPDH and miR-548ac genes

To confirm the specificity of amplification, we generated melting curves for each gene examined, as well as that of the endogenous GAPDH gene. By exploiting the first derivative of fluorescence, we were able to obtain a single predominant peak, testifying to the presence of a single type of amplification product. This attests to the specificity of the amplicons obtained and the absence of non-specific amplification products. These peaks appear at different melting temperatures (Tm), corresponding to the specific dissociation temperature of the amplification product for the detection of the Zeb1, GAPDH, miR-548ac, miR-101-1 and miR-96-5p genes, respectively. Note here the melting curve for the Zeb-1 gene (Figure 11).

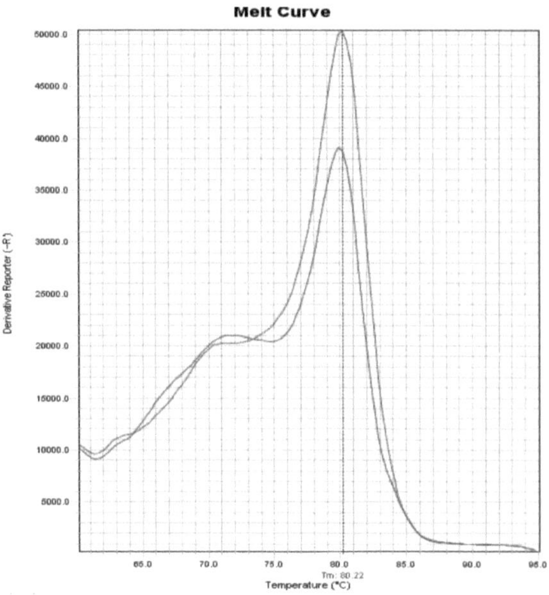

Figure 11: Zeb-1 gene melting curve

In a crucial step of our approach, we specifically targeted the evaluation of PCR E-efficiency. To this end, real-time PCR experiments were carried out on samples of increasing dilution in order to generate a standard curve representative of the primer pair dedicated to the locus of interest. This series of dilutions, notably with a factor of ½, should theoretically produce amplification curves shifted by one PCR cycle at each step, indicating an ideal reaction efficiency equal to 2, where the amount of DNA doubles at each cycle.

In this approach, the real-time PCR machine's built-in program was used to calculate the reaction's E-efficiency directly. Alternatively, real-time PCR was performed on a series of dilutions previously characterized by a known initial DNA quantity. These data were then positioned on a logarithmic scale graph, and the linear regression equation established across these points provided the reaction efficiency, identified by the directing coefficient of the regression line (Figure 12). This methodical approach ensured an accurate and reliable assessment of the efficiency of our PCR reaction.

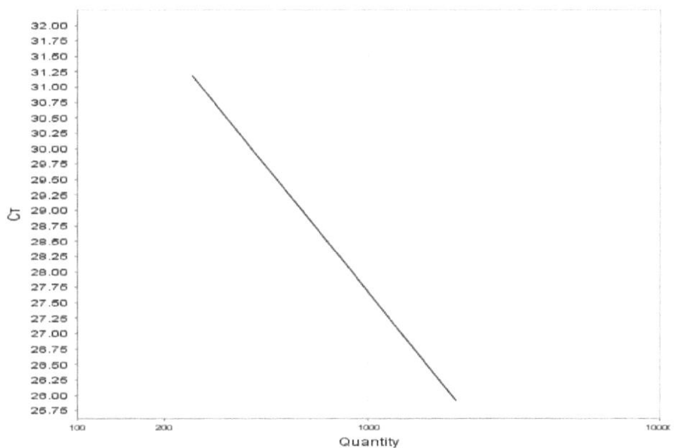

Figure 12: Efficiency or standard curve (Zeb-1 gene example)

III.   Expression profile of the Zeb-1 gene and 3 miRs

For the quantification of these markers we used real-time PCR specifically the Syber green method, and for the study of CF we adopted the relative method normalized by a calibrator (Benign Subject).

The results, expressed as FC, highlight significant overexpression of the Zeb-1 gene, miR-548ac and miR-96-5p in patients compared with healthy controls, with mean FCs of around 12.53, 5.42 and 158.13 respectively. However, with regard to miR-101, no distinction could be made between CP patients and benign controls (HR=1.3; p>0.05). This observation underlines a certain heterogeneity within the groups studied, suggesting a possible influence of patient-specific clinical and anatomopathological characteristics.

We then explored the possibility of a correlation between the expression levels of the three miRs (miR-548ac, miR-101-1 and miR-96-5p) and their target, Zeb-1.

Spearman's correlation was used for this purpose. The full results are summarized in Table 7, indicating the absence of any significant association between the miRs and their target, Zeb-1. However, a trend towards significance was observed, notably between miR-548ac and miR-96-5p on the one hand (p=0.075), and miR-96-5p and miR-101-1 on the other (p=0.071).

Table 7: Spearman correlation between Zeb-1 and miRs

			FC ZEB-1	FC miR-548ac	FC miR-101	FC-miR96
Spearm an's rho	FC ZEB-1	Correlation Coefficient	1,000	,327	,382	,111
		Sig. (2-tailed)	.	,234	,160	,694
		N	15	15	15	15
	FC miR-548ac	Correlation Coefficient	,327	1,000	,466	,474
		Sig. (2-tailed)	,234	.	,080	**,075**
		N	15	15	15	15
	FC miR-101	Correlation Coefficient	,382	,466	1,000	,479
		Sig. (2-tailed)	,160	,080	.	**,071**
		N	15	15	15	15
	FC-miR-96	Correlation Coefficient	,111	,474	,479	1,000
		Sig. (2-tailed)	,694	,075	,071	.
		N	15	15	15	15

To explore the association between Zeb-1, miR-548ac, miR-101-1 and miR-96-5p gene expression levels and clinico-pathological parameters such as disease stage and grade, as well as clinical parameters such as the presence of metastases, we employed the Kruskal-Wallis statistical test.

The distribution of Zeb-1 between the different stages, as illustrated in the box plot, shows great diversity among stage T2 patients, while the stage T1, T3 and T4 groups appear more homogeneous. Notable diversity was also observed within the T3 stage group when analyzing the distribution of miR-96-5p between the different stages. Furthermore, our results show that no significant association was demonstrated between the markers studied and the Gleason score. This lack of significant association with tumor grades was consistent, also manifesting itself in the analysis of other markers such as Zeb-1, miR-101-1 and miR-96-5p, with p-values of 0.28, 0.60 and 0.30 respectively.

Discussion

Prostate cancer is a multifactorial disease that progresses slowly in men over the age of 45. The etiology of this cancer remains enigmatic and unclear, despite scientific progress. Indeed, genetic studies have been multiplying over the last few years, with the aim of better understanding the molecular basis of prostate carcinogenesis and developing new prognostic markers. However, genetic approaches alone cannot explain the entire etiology of complex diseases, including prostate cancer.

In addition to the search for the effect of common or rare genetic variants, the search for secondary genetic effects should also be involved. These are effects that do not vary nucleotide sequences, but modulate gene expression. This is epigenetics, which represents a new aspect of cancer research. This mechanism involves DNA methylation, post-transcriptional histone modifications and the expression of miRs. These biomarkers attempt to predict the clinical evolution of cancer, enabling patients to be treated in an appropriate and personalized manner.

In the light of these data, we were interested in studying the expression profile of certain miRs and their targets which, according to the literature, appear to be most involved in the development of prostate cancer. To this end, we selected 3 miRs (miR-101-1, miR-548ac and miR-96-5p) that target a common gene called Zeb-1. A bioinformatics study combined with a literature search enabled us to choose this target gene in order to assess their regulation and impact on disease onset and progression. In this part of the project, we planned to carry out a study on a cohort of fresh tumors in order to understand the mechanisms of carcinogenesis and analyze the prognostic value of the markers studied. The chosen population consisted of some 35 fresh tumors, of which only 14 were retained for statistical analysis due to the poor quality of their RNAs. Two subjects with benign hyperplasia were used as controls in our analysis. The quality of the extracted

RNA molecules was checked on a Nanodrop to ensure that they were not degraded. The expression profile of these 3 miRs and of the Zeb-1 gene was established by the relative quantification method (double delta Ct method) using a calibration sample.

 In the first part, we studied the expression profiles of the Zeb-1 gene, mir-548ac, mir-101-1 and mir-96-5p. Statistical analysis, using Fold Change averaging, shows overexpression of the three markers Zeb-1, miR-548ac and miR-96-5p in prostate cancer patients compared with control subjects, with FC values of around 12.53, 5.42 and 158.13 respectively.

These results are both consistent with other work in the literature that has shown overexpression of the Zeb-1 gene, which showed that Zeb-1 expression was significantly increased in DU145 cells of the prostate cancer cell line (Lu et al., 2022; Orellana-Serradell, Herrera, Castellon, & Contreras, 2018). This overexpression has several consequences including enhanced cancer cell plasticity, which is considered an important driver of malignancy progression. The mechanism of Zeb-1-induced EMT relies on its binding to the promoter region of the epithelial cell marker protein E-cadherin, inhibiting its transcriptional expression and causing the loss of epithelial cell properties(Lu et al., 2022). Nancy et al. have shown in this context that the transcriptional factor Zeb-1 represses Syndecan 1 expression in prostate cancer. Syndecan 1 (SDC-1) is a cell-surface proteoglycan that plays an important role in cell adhesion, ensuring the maintenance of epithelial integrity, and its repression by Zeb-1 induces EMT (Farfán et al., 2018)..

Regarding the second marker, our study shows overexpression of miR-548ac which is in agreement with the study by Saffari et al. who showed overexpression of mir-548ac in cancerous samples and this expression further increases in high-grade prostate cancer compared to benign hyperplasia and normal tissue as non-cancerous tissue (Saffari et al., 2019). In this study mir-548ac acts as oncomiR by repressing PTEN expression. The tumor suppressor gene PTEN plays a key role in the regulation of the PI3k/AKT pathway, which is the most important signaling pathway that regulates certain cellular processes such as cell cycle, survival, metabolism, motility, genomic instability and angiogenesis and frequent changes in prostate cancer (Saffari et al., 2019). Rane JK et al. also showed that miR-548ac overexpression was confirmed in prostate cancer biopsies (five-fold, $p < 0.05$) and in unfractionated castration-resistant prostate cancers (1.8-fold, $p < 0.05$). An independent study showed that miR-548ac overexpression decreased doxorubicin-induced DNA damage in the cervical cancer cell line through inhibition of topoisomerase (DNA) II alpha 170kDa (TOP2A) (Rane et al., 2015). However, Shi Y et al, showed that miR-548ac was significantly under-expressed in breast cancer. Overexpression of miR-548 inhibited proliferation and promoted apoptosis in breast cancer cells. In addition, they demonstrated that the expression of ECHS1 (Enoyl Coenzyme A hydratase) involved in cell proliferation was significantly over-expressed in breast cancer cells and tissues; therefore, miR-548ac inhibits breast cancer cell proliferation by regulating ECHS1 expression.(Shi, Qiu, Wu, & Hai, 2015).

In the present work we also showed overexpression of the mir-96-5p gene, this result coincides with the findings of Haflidadóttir BS et al. who showed that miR-96-5p expression levels are elevated in prostate cancer (Haflidadóttir et al., 2013). Mir-96-5p is highly expressed in several other cancer types, including lymphoma, liver, breast, ovarian, lung, colon, testicular and colorectal cancer. MiR-96-5p has been suggested to act as an oncomiR regulating DNA proliferation and repair, but also as a tumor suppressor inducing apoptosis in pancreatic cells.

Secondly, in the case of miR-101-1, the CF value found cannot determine whether it is over- or underexpressed. These results do not seem to agree with the literature. Indeed, Lin et al. showed under-expression of miR-101-1 in prostate cancer biopsies compared with healthy controls (Lin et al., 2018). In other work, miR-101-1 has been reported underexpressed in gastric cancer, intrahepatic cholangiocarcinoma, osteosarcoma, hepatocellular carcinoma, non-small cell lung cancer, oral squamous cell carcinoma, transitional cell carcinoma of the bladder, cervical cancer, intraductal papillary mucinous neoplasm of the pancreas, breast cancer....etc (C. Z. Wang et al., 2018). Similarly, Varambally S, et al. and Chakravarthi et al. have shown that miR-101-1 is underexpressed in prostate cancer acting as a tumor suppressor via inhibition of EZH2 (Enhancer of zeste homolog 2 is a mammalian histone methyltransferase that contributes to epigenetic silencing of target genes and regulates cancer cell survival and metastasis)and SUB1(Transcriptional coactivator of RNA polymerase II) which promote metastasis(Chakravarthi et al., 2016; Varambally et al., 2008). This difference in miR-101-1 expression compared to our study suggests a certain heterogeneity within the groups, which could be explained by the clinical and anatomopathological characteristics of each patient studied. Hence the importance, on the one hand, of seeking correlation between markers and, on the other, of correlating molecular results with patients' clinical and anatomopathological parameters.

In the light of the results found, the distribution of expression of these 3 miRs and their target gene Zeb-1 in association with disease stages and grades shows no statistically significant difference. This was assessed by whisker curves and the Kruskal-Wallis test. These results are not in line with the literature. Indeed, Graham et al. have shown in a recent survey that Zeb-1 appears to be over-expressed in prostate cancer samples of high Gleason score compared with samples of lower malignancy (Graham et al., 2008). Similarly, Orellana S et al, have shown that Zeb-1 expression correlates with a Gleason score of >8 (Orellana-Serradell et al., 2018).. Concerning mir-548ac, Saffari et al. showed following qRT-PCR analysis that this marker was significantly increased in the Gleason score>7 group compared with the non-cancer group (*p < 0.05) (Saffari et al., 2019). For mir-96-5p, Haflidadóttir BS, et al, showed the association of this mir with a high Gleason score (>8) and high stage (T3, T4) (Haflidadóttir et al., 2013). With regard to mir-101-1, Lin et al. showed that underexpression of this mir is associated with a high Gleason score (Lin et al., 2018). This discrepancy in results between those found in this study, which showed that the expression level of our markers is associated with neither disease stage nor grade, and other work is mainly due to the small size of our cohort. In another stage, we set out to find an association between the markers Zeb-1, mir-548ac, mir-101-1 and mir-96-5p and the presence or absence of metastasis. To this end, patients were divided according to the presence or absence of metastasis. Based on the overall results and the "p" values, we have shown that there is no significant association between the presence or absence of metastasis and the CF of the various markers studied. These results are not, however, in line with the literature. Indeed, Jiawen Wu et al have shown that Zeb-1 promotes proliferation, invasion and metastasis in the DU145 prostate cancer cell line via suppression of the ERK1/2 signaling pathway and by promoting epithelial-mesenchymal transition through inhibition of E-Cadherin(Yang et al., 2020). Similarly, Nancy et al. have shown that Zeb-1 promotes metastasis by repressing Syndecan 1 expression in prostate cancer (Farfán et al., 2018).. Orellana S et al showed in the same context that Zeb-1 expression is higher in samples of higher malignancy and that Zeb-1 over-expression was able to induce epithelial-mesenchymal transition by up-regulating the mesenchymal marker Vimentin and down-regulating the epithelial marker E-Cadherin. In contrast, Zeb-1 inhibition repressed Vimentin expression and up-regulated E-Cadherin. Zeb-1 expression conferred higher motility, invasiveness and colony-forming capacity on 22Rv1 cells, whereas DU145 cells with Zeb-1 inhibition showed a decrease in these same properties. These results showed that Zeb-1 could be a key promoter of metastasis and tumor progression to advanced stages of prostate cancer. Several studies have shown that Zeb-1 in uterine, breast and other types of epithelial cancers is associated almost exclusively with the most aggressive classes, where its expression is linked to cell proliferation, invasion and metastasis (Orellana-Serradell et al., 2018). Concerning miR-548ac, Rane JK et al have shown that mir-548ac is associated with cell proliferation, invasion and metastasis and can be treated as a biomarker of progression in prostate cancer (Rane et al., 2015). Shi Y et al, demonstrated that miR-548ac inhibits the proliferation of breast cancer cells by regulating ECHS1 expression, indicating its potential as a therapeutic target for breast cancer (Shi et al., 2015). Haflidadóttir BS et al, showed that ectopic levels of miR-96-5p enhance cell growth and proliferation in prostate cancer cells, explaining that miR-96-5p has oncogenic properties and acts by decreasing levels of FOXO1 transcription and protein synthesis by binding to one of two predicted binding sites in the FOXO1 3'UTR sequence. Blocking this binding site completely inhibited the growth enhancement mediated by miR-96-5p. Taken together, these results indicate that miR-96-5p plays a key role in prostate cancer cell proliferation and may enhance prostate cancer progression. (Haflidadóttir et al., 2013). For mir 101-1, Lin et al, showed that this marker is predictive of metastasis in prostate cancer (Lin et al., 2018). Similarly, Varambally S, et al, showed that genomic loss of micro-101 leads to overexpression of histone methyltransferase EZH2 in prostate cancer. Enhancer of zeste homolog 2 (EZH2) is a mammalian histone methyltransferase that contributes to epigenetic silencing of target genes and regulates cancer cell survival and metastasis. EZH2 is overexpressed in aggressive solid tumors by mechanisms that remain unclear. Here, Varambally S, et al, have shown that EZH2 expression and function in cancer cell lines are inhibited by mir-101. Analysis of human prostate tumours revealed that miR-101-1 expression decreases during cancer progression, in parallel with an increase in EZH2 expression, resulting in tumour progression, cell proliferation, colony formation and increased invasion (Varambally et al., 2008).

In conclusion, and in the light of these results, which seem to be limited by the small number of participants, we have the impression that our results are sometimes at odds with other studies. We therefore suggest continuing to collect biological material in order to improve the efficiency of the statistical tests and thus find good results that are consistent with those published in the literature. We are also keen to analyze other markers that could play an important role in prostate carcinogenesis, in conjunction with the microRNAs selected in this work. In addition, the functional part of the study seems to be equally important for understanding the mechanisms of epigenetic regulation of this cancer.

Conclusion and outlook

In the context of targeted therapy, epigenetics seems to be one of the most promising avenues for cancer treatment in recent years. The search for new markers capable of improving the prognosis and diagnosis of patients is becoming essential. Among epigenetic mechanisms, microRNAs play a major role in cancer diseases such as prostate cancer.

In this work, our choice was based on the selection of markers most implicated in the occurrence of prostate tumors. The Zeb-1 gene is involved in several cellular processes, especially the epithelial-mesenchymal transition, which plays an essential role in tumor invasion. Zeb-1 can directly or indirectly suppress the expression of E-cadherin, an important inhibitor of EMT. This inhibition has a number of consequences on cancer, notably promoting cell proliferation and invasion, as well as metastasis. In this context, we analyzed tumor samples from prostate cancer patients obtained following resection of prostate tumors. These samples were provided by the Urology Department of Charles Nicolle Hospital, Tunis. We first quantified the level of zeb-1 gene expression in tumor tissue compared with healthy controls by RT-qPCR. Our results, based solely on 14 patients, showed that this gene is over-expressed in tumors compared with normal tissue. We then set out to determine the epigenetic mechanisms responsible for deregulation of the zeb-1 gene in prostate cancer. Based on literature data, deregulation of Zeb-1 gene expression in prostate cancer may be due to deregulation of microRNA expression. We identified by in silico analysis that mir-548ac, mir-101-1 and mir-96-5p seem to be among the potential targets of Zeb-1. For this reason, we analyzed the expression levels of mir-548ac, mir-101-1 and mir-96-5p in tumor versus healthy tissue in the same way as the Zeb-1 gene. The mean Fold Change values found in the same cohort show over-expression of mir-548ac and mir-96-5p in tumors versus normal tissue, while no conclusions can be drawn regarding mir-101 expression. This suggests a kind of heterogeneity within the groups, which could be explained by the clinical and anatomopathological characteristics of each patient. Hence the importance, in the second part of this work, of correlating the molecular results of the markers studied with the clinical and anatomopathological parameters of the patients. To this end, we correlated our markers according to stages T1, T2, T3 and T4 of the disease. The whisker curves obtained, confirmed by the Kruskal-Wallis test, show no statistically significant difference between tumor stage and marker expression, as demonstrated by the p-values obtained.

In another part of this work, we studied the correlation between the expression of the same markers and the grade of the disease. This analysis is based on the Gleason score. As a result, the whisker curves and the Krustal-Wallis test show no significant differences between expression and tumor grade.

The final stage of this study involved the search for a possible association between the markers studied and the presence or absence of a metastasis. To this end, patients were classified according to the presence or absence of metastasis. Our results on 14 patients showed no statistically significant difference between the presence of a metastasis and the CF of the various markers.

The search for a correlation between Zeb-1 and the 3 mirs studied was among our main objectives in order to understand epigenetic deregulation between a microRNA and its target. The Spearman correlation showed no significant association. However, a trend towards significance was observed between mir-548ac and mir-96-5p on the one hand (p=0.075) and mir-96-5p and mir-101-1 on the other (p=0.071). This suggests that the 3 mirs do not control the expression level of the Zeb-1 gene. Several hypotheses can be put forward, such as the small size of the study cohort, presumably insufficient for proper statistical analysis, or the involvement of other microRNAs in the regulation of Zeb-1 expression in patients with prostatic adenocarcinoma.

In the future, we plan to increase the size of our study population, a limiting factor in this work, which must also be heterogeneous. Indeed, the lack of correlation between Zeb-1 expression and mirs needs to be verified by functional and proteomic analyses. We also plan to investigate other genetic and epi-genetic alterations that could explain the deregulation of the zeb-1 gene in prostate cancer. In addition, long-term follow-up of patients is required before any conclusions can be drawn.

References

1. Bray F., Ferlay J., Soerjomataram I., Siegel R. L., Torre L. A. & Jemal A. 2018 Global cancer statistics 2018: GLOBOCAN estimates of incidence and mortality worldwide for 36 cancers in 185 countries. *CA: A Cancer Journal for Clinicians.* **68,** 394-424.

2. Lee, C. H., O. Akin-Olugbade and A. Kirschenbaum (2011). "Overview of prostate anatomy, histology, and pathology." Endocrinol Metab Clin North Am 40(3): 565-575, viii-ix.

3. Toivanen, R. and M. M. Shen (2017). "Prostate organogenesis: tissue induction, hormonal regulation and cell type specification." Development 144(8): 1382-1398.

4. McNeal, J. E. (1981). "The zonal anatomy of the prostate." Prostate 2(1): 35-49.

5. McNeal, J. E. (1988). "Normal histology of the prostate." Am J Surg Pathol 12(8): 619-633.

6. Briganti, A., U. Capitanio, N. Suardi, A. Gallina, A. Salonia, M. Bianchi, M. Tutolo, V. Di Girolamo, G. Guazzoni, P. Rigatti and F. Montorsi (2009). "Benign Prostatic Hyperplasia and Its Aetiologies." European Urology Supplements 8(13): 865-871.

7. Barry, M. J., F. J. Fowler, Jr, P. O'Leary M, R. C. Bruskewitz, H. L. Holtgrewe, W.K. Mebust and A. T. Cockett (2017). "The American Urological Association Symptom Index for Benign Prostatic Hyperplasia." J Urol 197(2s): S189-s197.

8. Hall, W. C., S. W. Nielsen and K. McEntee (1976). "Tumours of the prostate and penis." Bulletin of the World Health Organization 53(2-3): 247-256.

9. Vrubel, F., J. Mraz, R. Nemecek, F. Papousek and M. Hanselova (1979). "Carcinoma of the prostate. I. Histochemical examination as an aid in evaluating prostate carcinoma." Int Urol Nephrol 11(4): 295-299. Siegel RL, Miller KD, Jemal A (2017) Cancer statistics, 2017. CA 67(1):7-30. https://doi.org/10.3322/caac.21387.

10. Fournier, G., A. Valeri, P. Mangin and O. Cussenot (2004). "Prostate cancer. Treatment." Annales d'Urologie 38(5): 225-258.

11. Castillejos-Molina, R. A. and F. B. Gabilondo-Navarro (2016). "Prostate cancer." Salud Publica Mex 58(2): 279-284.

12. Norgaard, M., A. O. Jensen, J. B. Jacobsen, K. Cetin, J. P. Fryzek and H. T. Sorensen (2010). "Skeletal related events, bone metastasis and survival of prostate cancer: a population based cohort study in Denmark (1999 to 2007)." J Urol 184(1): 162-167.

13. Keto CJ, Freedland SJA, Risk-Stratified Approach to prostate- specific antigen screening. Eur Urol 59(4):506-508. https://doi. org/10.1016/j.eururo.2011.01.029

14. Rozet, F., C. Hennequin, J. B. Beauval, P. Beuzeboc, L. Cormier, G. Fromont, P. Mongiat-Artus, A. Ouzzane, G. Ploussard, D. Azria, I. Brenot-Rossi, G. Cancel-Tassin, O. Cussenot, T. Lebret, X. Rebillard, M. Soulie, R. Renard-Penna and A. Mejean (2016). "[CCAFU french national guidelines 2016-2018 on prostate cancer]." <u>Prog Urol</u> **27 Suppl 1**: S95-s143.

15. Leitzmann, M. F., E. A. Platz, M. J. Stampfer, W. C. Willett and E. Giovannucci (2004). "Ejaculation frequency and subsequent risk of prostate cancer." <u>Jama</u> **291**(13): 1578-1586

16. Daniyal, M., Z. A. Siddiqui, M. Akram, H. M. Asif, S. Sultana and A. Khan (2014). "Epidemiology, etiology, diagnosis and treatment of prostate cancer." <u>Asian Pac J Cancer Prev</u> **15**(22): 9575-9578.

17. Alexander, D. D., P. J. Mink, C. A. Cushing and B. Sceurman (2010). "A review and meta-analysis of prospective studies of red and processed meat intake and prostate cancer." <u>Nutr J</u> **9**: 50.

18. Leitzmann, M. F. and S. Rohrmann (2012). "Risk factors for the onset of prostatic cancer: age, location, and behavioral correlates." <u>Clin Epidemiol</u> **4**: 1-11.

19. Giovannucci, E. A. Platz, S. Sutcliffe, K. Fall, T. Kurth, J. Ma, M. J. Stampfer and L. A. Mucci (2009). "Prospective study of Trichomonas vaginalis infection and prostate cancer incidence and mortality: Physicians' Health Study." <u>Journal of the National Cancer Institute</u> **101**(20): 1406-1411.

20. Antonelli, J., S. J. Freedland and L. W. Jones (2009). "Exercise therapy across the prostate cancer continuum." <u>Prostate Cancer And Prostatic Diseases</u> **12**: 110.

21. Parent, M.-E., M. Désy and J. Siemiatycki (2009). "Does exposure to agricultural chemicals increase the risk of prostate cancer among farmers?" <u>McGill journal of medicine: MJM: an international forum for the advancement of medical sciences by students</u> **12**(1): 70-77.

22. Michaud, D. S., S. E. Daugherty, S. I. Berndt, E. A. Platz, M. Yeager, E. D. Crawford, A. Hsing, W.-Y. Huang and R. B. Hayes (2006). "Genetic polymorphisms of interleukin-1B (IL-1B), IL-6, IL-8, and IL-10 and risk of prostate cancer." <u>Cancer research</u> **66**(8): 4525-4530.

23. Yao, S., C. Till, A. R. Kristal, P. J. Goodman, A. W. Hsing, C. M. Tangen, E. A. Platz, F. Z. Stanczyk, J. K. V. Reichardt, L. Tang, M. L. Neuhouser, R. M. Santella,

W. D. Figg, D. K. Price, H. L. Parnes, S. M. Lippman, I. M. Thompson, C. B. Ambrosone and A. Hoque (2011). "Serum estrogen levels and prostate cancer risk in the prostate cancer prevention trial: a nested case-control study." Cancer causes & control: CCC 22(8): 1121- 1131.

24. Sutcliffe Yegnasubramanian, S., J. Kowalski, M. L. Gonzalgo, M. Zahurak, S. Piantadosi, P. C. Walsh, G. S. Bova, A. M. De Marzo, W. B. Isaacs and W. G. Nelson (2004). "Hypermethylation of CpG islands in primary and metastatic human prostate cancer." Cancer Res 64(6): 1975-1986.

25. Stark, J. R., G. Judson, J. F. Alderete, V. Mundodi, A. S. Kucknoor, E. L. Giovannucci, E. A. Platz, S. Sutcliffe, K. Fall, T. Kurth, J. Ma, M. J. Stampfer and L. A. Mucci (2009). "Prospective study of Trichomonas vaginalis infection and prostate cancer incidence and mortality: Physicians' Health Study." Journal of the National Cancer Institute 101(20): 1406-1411.

26. Cheng, I., J. S. Witte, S. J. Jacobsen, R. Haque, V. P. Quinn, C. P. Quesenberry, B. J. Caan and S. K. Van Den Eeden (2010). "Prostatitis, sexually transmitted diseases, and prostate cancer: the California Men's Health Study." PLoS One 5(1): e8736.

27. Leitzmann, M. F., E. A. Platz, M. J. Stampfer, W. C. Willett and E. Giovannucci (2004). "Ejaculation frequency and subsequent risk of prostate cancer." Jama 291(13): 1578-1586 .

28. Murata, M., M. Watanabe, M. Yamanaka, Y. Kubota, H. Ito, M. Nagao, T. Katoh, T. Kamataki, J. Kawamura, R. Yatani and T. Shiraishi (2001). "Genetic polymorphisms in cytochrome P450 (CYP) 1A1, CYP1A2, CYP2E1, glutathione S-transferase (GST) M1 and GSTT1 and susceptibility to prostate cancer in the Japanese population." Cancer Lett 165(2): 171-177.

29. Murata, T., K. Takayama, T. Urano, T. Fujimura, D. Ashikari, D. Obinata, K. Horie- Inoue, S. Takahashi, Y. Ouchi, Y. Homma and S. Inoue (2012). "14-3-3 , a Novel Androgen-Responsive Gene, Is Upregulated in Prostate Cancer and Promotes Prostate Cancer Cell Proliferation and Survival." Clinical cancer research : an official journal of the American Association for Cancer Research 18: 5617- 5627.

30. Hirata H, Hinoda Y, Tanaka Y, Okayama N, Suehiro Y, Kawa- moto K, Kikuno N, Majid S, Vejdani K, Dahiya R (2007) Poly- morphisms of DNA repair genes are risk factors for prostate cancer. Eur J Cancer (Oxford, England 1990)

43(2):231-237. https://doi.org/10.1016/j.ejca.2006.11.005

31. Nakagawa, H., S. Akamatsu and R. Takata (2016). "[Genome-wide association study(GWAS) and genetic risk of prostate cancer]." Nihon rinsho. Japanese journal of clinical medicine 74(1): 34-39.

32. Benafif Naylor, S. L. (2007). "SNPs associated with prostate cancer risk and prognosis." Front Biosci 12: 4111-4131.

33. Collin, S. M., C. Metcalfe, L. Zuccolo, S. J. Lewis, L. Chen, A. Cox, M. Davis, J. A. Lane, J. Donovan, G. D. Smith, D. E. Neal, F. C. Hamdy, J. Gudmundsson, P. Sulem, T. Rafnar, K. R. Benediktsdottir, R. A. Eeles, M. Guy, Z. Kote-Jarai, J. Morrison, A.

34. Choi, J. Y., M. L. Neuhouser, M. J. Barnett, C. C. Hong, A. R. Kristal, M. D. Thornquist, I. B. King, G. E. Goodman and C. B. Ambrosone (2008). "Iron intake, oxidative stress-related genes (MnSOD and MPO) and prostate cancer risk in CARET cohort." Carcinogenesis 29(5): 964-970.

35. Rybicki, B. A., D. V. Conti, A. Moreira, M. Cicek, G. Casey and J. S. Witte (2004). "DNA repair gene XRCC1 and XPD polymorphisms and risk of prostate cancer." Cancer Epidemiol Biomarkers Prev 13(1): 23-29.

36. Hirata H, Hinoda Y, Tanaka Y, Okayama N, Suehiro Y, Kawa- moto K, Kikuno N, Majid S, Vejdani K, Dahiya R (2007) Poly- morphisms of DNA repair genes are risk factors for prostate cancer. Eur J Cancer (Oxford, England 1990) 43(2):231-237. https://doi.org/10.1016/j.ejca.2006.11.005

37. Schoenborn, J. R., P. Nelson and M. Fang (2013). "Genomic profiling defines subtypes of prostate cancer with the potential for therapeutic stratification." Clin Cancer Res 19(15): 4058-4066.

38. Shindo, T., H. Kurihara, K. Kuno, H. Yokoyama, T. Wada, Y. Kurihara, T. Imai, Y. Wang, M. Ogata, H. Nishimatsu, N. Moriyama, Y. Oh-hashi, H. Morita, T. Ishikawa, R. Nagai, Y. Yazaki and K. Matsushima (2000). "ADAMTS-1: a metalloproteinase- disintegrin essential for normal growth, fertility, and organ morphology and function." J Clin Invest 105(10): 1345-1352.

39. Shindo, T., H. Kurihara, K. Kuno, H. Yokoyama, T. Wada, Y. Kurihara, T. Imai, Y. Wang, M. Ogata, H. Nishimatsu, N. Moriyama, Y. Oh-hashi, H. Morita, T. Ishikawa, R. Nagai, Y. Yazaki and K. Matsushima (2000). "ADAMTS-1: a metalloproteinase- disintegrin essential for normal growth, fertility, and organ morphology and function." J Clin Invest 105(10): 1345-1352.

40. Gustavsson, H., W. Wang, K. Jennbacken, K. Welen and J. E. Damber (2009). "ADAMTS1, a putative anti-angiogenic factor, is decreased in human prostate cancer." BJU Int 104(11): 1786-1790.

41. Obsil, T. and V. Obsilova (2008). "Structure/function relationships underlying regulation of FOXO transcription factors." Oncogene 27(16): 2263-2275.

42. Huang, F., X. Li, Q. Du and X. Zhang (2018). "[Expression of forkhead transcription factor O4 in prostate cancer and its effect on prostate cancer cell invasion]." Zhong Nan Da Xue Xue Bao Yi Xue Ban 43(11): 1194-1201.

43. Zennami, K., S. M. Choi, R. Liao, Y. Li, W. Dinalankara, L. Marchionni, F. H. Rafiqi, A. Kurozumi, K. Hatano and S. E. Lupold (2019). "PDCD4 Is an Androgen- Repressed Tumor Suppressor that Regulates Prostate Cancer Growth and Castration Resistance." Mol Cancer Res 17(2): 618-627.

44. Heard, E. and R. A. Martienssen (2014). "Transgenerational epigenetic inheritance: myths and mechanisms." Cell 157(1): 95-109.

45. Kyburz, D., E. Karouzakis and C. Ospelt (2014). "Epigenetic changes: the missing link." Best Pract Res Clin Rheumatol 28(4): 577-587.

46. Moore, L. D., T. Le and G. Fan (2013). "DNA methylation and its basic function." Neuropsychopharmacology 38(1): 23-38.

47. Jin, B., Y. Li and K. D. Robertson (2011). "DNA methylation: superior or subordinate in the epigenetic hierarchy?" Genes Cancer 2(6): 607-617.

48. Graff, J. R., J. G. Herman, R. G. Lapidus, H. Chopra, R. Xu, D. F. Jarrard, W. B. Isaacs, P. M. Pitha, N. E. Davidson and S. B. Baylin (1995). "E-cadherin expression is silenced by DNA hypermethylation in human breast and prostate carcinomas." Cancer Res 55(22): 5195-5199.

49. Cairns, P., M. Esteller, J. G. Herman, M. Schoenberg, C. Jeronimo, M. Sanchez-Cespedes, N. H. Chow, M. Grasso, L. Wu, W. B. Westra and D. Sidransky (2001). "Molecular detection of prostate cancer in urine by GSTP1 hypermethylation." Clin Cancer Res 7(9): 2727-2730.

50. Yan, H., S. Wang, H. Yu, J. Zhu and C. Chen (2013). "Molecular pathways and functional analysis of miRNA expression associated with paclitaxel-induced apoptosis in hepatocellular carcinoma cells." Pharmacology 92(3-4): 167-174.

51. Zhao, F., E. Olkhov-Mitsel, S. Kamdar, R. Jeyapala, J. Garcia, R. Hurst, M. Y. Hanna, R. Mills, A. V. Tuzova, E. O'Reilly, S. Kelly, C. Cooper, D. Brewer, A. S. Perry J. Clark, N. Fleshner and B. Bapat (2018). "A urine-based DNA methylation assay, ProCUrE, to

identify clinically significant prostate cancer." <u>Clin Epigenetics</u> **10**(1): 147. Abbas, A. and S. Gupta (2008). "The role of histone deacetylases in prostate cancer." <u>Epigenetics</u> **3**(6): 300-309.

52. Collin Ngollo, M., A. Dagdemir, S. Karsli-Ceppioglu, G. Judes, A. Pajon, F. Penault-Llorca, J. P. Boiteux, Y. J. Bignon, L. Guy and D. J. Bernard-Gallon (2014). "Epigenetic modifications in prostate cancer." <u>Epigenomics</u> **6**(4): 415-426.

53. Kyburz, D., E. Karouzakis and C. Ospelt (2014). "Epigenetic changes: the missing link." <u>Best Pract Res Clin Rheumatol</u> **28**(4): 577-587.

54. Chou, C. H., S. Shrestha, C. D. Yang, N. W. Chang, Y. L. Lin, K. W. Liao, W. C. Huang, T. H. Sun, S. J. Tu, W. H. Lee, M. Y. Chiew, C. S. Tai, T. Y. Wei, T. R. Tsai, H. T. Huang, C. Y. Wang, H. Y. Wu, S. Y. Ho, P. R. Chen, C. H. Chuang, P. J. Hsieh, Y. S. Wu, W. L. Chen, M. J. Li, Y. C. Wu, X. Y. Huang, F. L. Ng, W. Buddhakosai, P. C. Huang, K. C. Lan, C. Y. Huang, S. L. Weng, Y. N. Cheng, C. Liang, W. L. Hsu and H. D. Huang (2018). "miRTarBase update 2018: a resource for experimentally validated microRNA-target interactions." Nucleic Acids Res 46(D1): D296-d302.

55. Bartels, C. L. and G. J. Tsongalis (2009). "MicroRNAs: novel biomarkers for human cancer." <u>Clin Chem</u> **55**(4): 623-631.

56. Lai, E. C. (2002). "Micro RNAs are complementary to 3' UTR sequence motifs that mediate negative post-transcriptional regulation." <u>Nat Genet</u> **30**(4): 363-364.

57. Mohr, A. M. and J. L. Mott (2015). "Overview of MicroRNA Biology." <u>Semin Liver Dis</u> **35**(01): 003-011.

58. Morgan, C. P. and T. L. Bale (2012). "Sex differences in microRNA regulation of gene expression: no smoke, just miRs." <u>Biology of Sex Differences</u> **3**(1): 22.

59. Iorio, M. V. and C. M. Croce (2012). "microRNA involvement in human cancer." <u>Carcinogenesis</u> **33**(6): 1126-1133.

60. Vanacore, D., M. Boccellino, S. Rossetti, C. Cavaliere, C. D'Aniello, R. Di Franco, F. J. Romano, M. Montanari, E. La Mantia, R. Piscitelli, F. Nocerino, F. Cappuccio, G. Grimaldi, A. Izzo, L. Castaldo, M. F. Pepe, M. G. Malzone, G. Iovane, G. Ametrano, P. Stiuso, L. Quagliuolo, D. Barberio, S. Perdona, P. Muto, M. Montella, P. Maiolino, B. M. Veneziani, G. Botti, M. Caraglia and G. Facchini (2017). "Micrornas in prostate cancer: an overview." Oncotarget 8(30): 50240-50251.

61. Srikok, S., P. Chuammitri and Cmvj (2016). "MicroRNAs as a potential biomarker

in bovine mastitis." Chiang Mai Veterinary Journal 14: 1-12.

62. Wu, X. and J. Gu (2016). "Heritability of prostate cancer: a tale of rare variants and common single nucleotide polymorphisms." Ann Transl Med 4(10): 206.

63. Benafif, S., Z. Kote-Jarai, R. A. Eeles and P. Consortium (2018). "A Review of Prostate Cancer Genome-Wide Association Studies (GWAS)." Cancer epidemiology, biomarkers & prevention: a publication of the American Association for Cancer Research, cosponsored by the American Society of Preventive Oncology 27(8): 845- 857.

64. Cybulski, C. (2007). "Selected aspects of inherited susceptibility to prostate cancer and tumours of different site of origin." Hered Cancer Clin Pract 5(3): 164-179.

65. Mao, G. E., V. E. Reuter, C. Cordon-Cardo, G. Dalbagni, H. I. Scher, J. B. DeKernion, Z. F. Zhang and J. Rao (2004). "Decreased retinoid X receptor-alpha protein expression in basal cells occurs in the early stage of human prostate cancer development." Cancer Epidemiol Biomarkers Prev 13(3): 383-390.

66. Higuchi, T., M. Nakamura, K. Shimada, E. Ishida, K. Hirao and N. Konishi (2008). "HRK inactivation associated with promoter methylation and LOH in prostate cancer." Prostate 68(1): 105-113.

67. Hu, X. Y., Y. M. Xu, X. C. Chen, H. Ping, Z. H. Chen and F. Q. Zeng (2006). "Immunohistochemical analysis of Omi/HtrA2 expression in prostate cancer and benign prostatic hyperplasia." Apmis 114(12): 893-898.

68. Higuchi, T., M. Nakamura, K. Shimada, E. Ishida, K. Hirao and N. Konishi (2008). "HRK inactivation associated with promoter methylation and LOH in prostate cancer." Prostate 68(1): 105-113.

69. Dhillon, P. K., M. Barry, M. J. Stampfer, S. Perner, M. Fiorentino, A. Fornari, J. Ma, J. Fleet, T. Kurth, M. A. Rubin and L. A. Mucci (2009). "Aberrant cytoplasmic expression of p63 and prostate cancer mortality." Cancer epidemiology, biomarkers & prevention: a publication of the American Association for Cancer Research, cosponsored by the American Society of Preventive Oncology 18(2): 595-600.

70. Wong, A. K., Y. Chen, L. Lian, P. C. Ha, K. Petersen, K. Laity, A. Carillo, M. Emerson, K. Heichman, J. Gupte, S. V. Tavtigian and D. H. Teng (1999). "Genomic structure, chromosomal location, and mutation analysis of the human CDC14A gene." Genomics 59(2): 248-251.

71. Chakravarthi, B. V., Goswami, M. T., Pathi, S. S., Robinson, A. D., Cieślik, M.,

Chandrashekar, D. S., . . . Varambally, S. (2016). MicroRNA-101 regulated transcriptional modulator SUB1 plays a role in prostate cancer. Oncogene, 35(49), 6330-6340. doi:10.1038/onc.2016.164

72. Farfán, N., Ocarez, N., Castellón, E. A., Mejía, N., de Herreros, A. G., & Contreras, H. R. (2018). The transcriptional factor ZEB1 represses Syndecan 1 expression in prostate cancer. Sci Rep, 8(1), 11467. doi:10.1038/s41598-018-29829-1

73. Graham, T. R., Zhau, H. E., Odero-Marah, V. A., Osunkoya, A. O., Kimbro, K. S., Tighiouart, M., . . . O'Regan, R. M. (2008). Insulin-like growth factor-I-dependent up-regulation of ZEB1 drives epithelial-to-mesenchymal transition in human prostate cancer cells. Cancer Res, 68(7), 2479-2488. doi:10.1158/0008-5472.can-07-2559

74. Haflidadóttir, B. S., Larne, O., Martin, M., Persson, M., Edsjö, A., Bjartell, A., & Ceder, Y. (2013). Upregulation of miR-96 enhances cellular proliferation of prostate cancer cells through FOXO1. PLoS One, 8(8), e72400. doi:10.1371/journal.pone.0072400

75. Lin, Y., Chen, F., Shen, L., Tang, X., Du, C., Sun, Z., ... Shen, B. (2018). Biomarker microRNAs for prostate cancer metastasis: screened with a network vulnerability analysis model. Journal of Translational Medicine, 16(1), 134. doi:10.1186/s12967-018-1506-7

76. Lu, J., Fei, F., Wu, C., Mei, J., Xu, J., & Lu, P. (2022). ZEB1: Catalyst of immune escape during tumor metastasis. Biomedicine & Pharmacotherapy, 153, 113490. doi:https://doi.org/10.1016/j.biopha.2022.113490

77. Madany, M., Thomas, T., & Edwards, L. A. (2018). The Curious Case of ZEB1. Discoveries (Craiova), 6(4), e86. doi:10.15190/d.2018.7

78. Orellana-Serradell, O., Herrera, D., Castellon, E. A., & Contreras, H. R. (2018). The transcription factor ZEB1 promotes an aggressive phenotype in prostate cancer cell lines. Asian J Androl, 20(3), 294-299. doi:10.4103/aja.aja_61_17

79. Perez-Oquendo, M., & Gibbons, D. L. (2022). Regulation of ZEB1 Function and Molecular Associations in Tumor Progression and Metastasis. Cancers (Basel), 14(8). doi:10.3390/cancers14081864

80. Rane, J. K., Scaravilli, M., Ylipää, A., Pellacani, D., Mann, V. M., Simms, M. S., . . . Maitland, N. J. (2015). MicroRNA expression profile of primary prostate cancer stem cells as a source of biomarkers and therapeutic targets. Eur Urol, 67(1), 7-10. doi:10.1016/j.eururo.2014.09.005

81. Ribatti, D., Tamma, R., & Annese, T. (2020). Epithelial-Mesenchymal Transition in Cancer: A Historical Overview. Translational Oncology, 13(6), 100773. doi:https://doi.org/10.1016/j.tranon.2020.100773

82. Roche, J. (2018). The Epithelial-to-Mesenchymal Transition in Cancer. Cancers (Basel), 10(2). doi:10.3390/cancers10020052

83. Saffari, M., Ghaderian, S. M. H., Omrani, M. D., Afsharpad, M., Shankaie, K., & Samadaian, N. (2019). The Association of miR-let 7b and miR-548 with PTEN in Prostate Cancer. Urol J, 16(3), 267-273. doi:10.22037/uj.v0i0.4564

84. Sharma, P. C., & Gupta, A. (2020). MicroRNAs: potential biomarkers for diagnosis and prognosis of different cancers. Translational Cancer Research, 9(9), 5798-5818.

85. Shi, Y., Qiu, M., Wu, Y., & Hai, L. (2015). MiR-548-3p functions as an anti-oncogenic regulator in breast cancer. Biomed Pharmacother, 75, 111-116. doi:10.1016/j.biopha.2015.07.027

86. Varambally, S., Cao, Q., Mani, R. S., Shankar, S., Wang, X., Ateeq, B., . . . Chinnaiyan, A. M. (2008). Genomic loss of microRNA-101 leads to overexpression of histone methyltransferase EZH2 in cancer. Science, 322(5908), 1695-1699. doi:10.1126/science.1165395

87. Wang, C., Lu, S., Jiang, J., Jia, X., Dong, X., & Bu, P. (2014). Hsa-microRNA-101 suppresses migration and invasion by targeting Rac1 in thyroid cancer cells. Oncol Lett, 8(4), 1815-1821. doi:10.3892/ol.2014.2361

88. Wang, C. Z., Deng, F., Li, H., Wang, D. D., Zhang, W., Ding, L., & Tang, J. H. (2018). MiR-101: a potential therapeutic target of cancers. Am J Transl Res, 10(11), 3310-3321.

89. Wang, H., Ma, N., Li, W., & Wang, Z. (2020). MicroRNA-96-5p promotes proliferation, invasion and EMT of oral carcinoma cells by directly targeting FOXF2. Biol Open, 9(3). doi:10.1242/bio.049478

90. Yang, C., Li, Q., Chen, X., Zhang, Z., Mou, Z., Ye, F., ... Jiang, H. (2020). Circular RNA circRGNEF promotes bladder cancer progression via miR-548/KIF2C axis regulation. Aging (Albany NY), 12(8), 6865-6879. doi:10.18632/aging.103047

91. Zhang, Y., Xu, L., Li, A., & Han, X. (2019). The roles of ZEB1 in tumorigenic progression and epigenetic modifications. Biomedicine & Pharmacotherapy, 110, 400-408. doi:https://doi.org/10.1016/j.biopha.2018.11.112

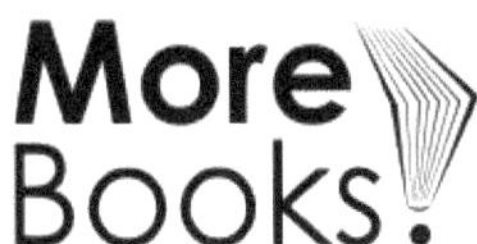

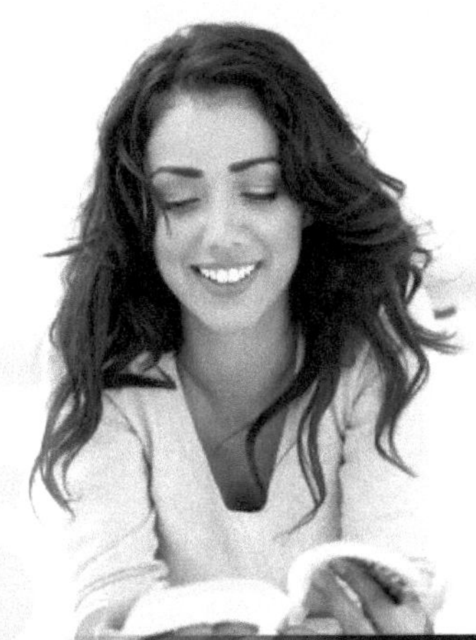

I want morebooks!

Buy your books fast and straightforward online - at one of world's fastest growing online book stores! Environmentally sound due to Print-on-Demand technologies.

Buy your books online at
www.morebooks.shop

Kaufen Sie Ihre Bücher schnell und unkompliziert online – auf einer der am schnellsten wachsenden Buchhandelsplattformen weltweit! Dank Print-On-Demand umwelt- und ressourcenschonend produziert.

Bücher schneller online kaufen
www.morebooks.shop

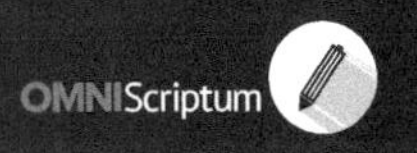

info@omniscriptum.com
www.omniscriptum.com

OMNIScriptum

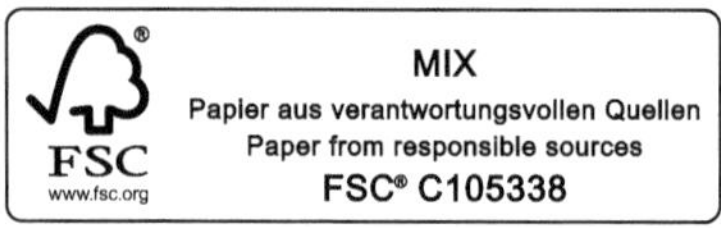

Printed by Books on Demand GmbH, Norderstedt / Germany